# HAEMOSTATIC DRUGS
## A critical appraisal

«The change from clinical impressions and impressionable physicians to the measurement of the probability of accuracy in clinical observations and medical research, have been the areas of greatest advance. Statements of opinion now require statistical support if they are to command clinical backing and action».

W.S. PEART in the foreword to *Medical Research*, J.M. England, Churchill Livingstone, 1975.

# HAEMOSTATIC DRUGS

## A critical appraisal

M. VERSTRAETE

M.D. (Leuven), F.R.C.P. (Edin.),
F.A.C.P. (Hon.); Professor of Medi-
cine; Director, Laboratory of Blood
Coagulation, Department of Medical
Research, University of Leuven.

In collaboration with B. Bennett (Aberdeen), M. Brozović (London),
D. Collen (Leuven), G. de Gaetano (Milano), M. N. G. Dukes (The Hague),
P. T. Flute (London), P. J. Gaffney (London), S. Garattini (Milano),
J. Hugues (Liège), K. Lechner (Wien), R. Masure (Brussels), G. P. McNicol
(Leeds), I. M. Nilsson (Malmö), L. Poller (Manchester), C. R. M. Prentice
(Glasgow), J. Roos (The Hague), A. A. Sharp (Oxford), J. J. Sixma
(Utrecht), J. van de Loo (Münster), K. W. von Eickstedt (Berlin),
J. Vermylen (Leuven), J. L. Wautier (Paris)

MARTINUS NIJHOFF MEDICAL DIVISION THE HAGUE 1977

ISBN-13: 978-90-247-2020-0    e-ISBN-13: 978-94-010-1106-8
DOI: 10.1007/978-94-010-1106-8

© 1977. Martinus Nijhoff, P.O.B. 442, The Hague, The Netherlands.

Softcover reprint of the hardcover 1st edition 1977

# Background for a critical review of general haemostatic drugs

The control of spontaneous and postoperative haemorrhage is a matter of concern particularly to surgeons, anaesthetists, haematologists and the patient. In some instances the control of bleeding may be relatively simple using some topical therapeutic procedure or specific correction of the haemostatic defect. On other occasions the patient's course may dictate more radical and even life-saving measures. In either situation, any therapeutic agent which facilitates control of haemorrhage is a welcome addition to the therapeutic armament.

Besides some vitamins, blood products and agents for topical use, there are only a few agents with a well-defined action on the haemostatic mechanism, which are of proven clinical value in bleeding patients. In contrast, a rather large number of drugs are being marketed as haemostatic agents for the treatment of bleeding disorders or the prevention of haemorrhage. It was felt that the time had come to study in detail the validity of the clinical evidence on which these agents are recommended for the treatment of bleeding disorders.

To this end a symposium was organised at the University of Leuven on May 28-29th 1976, on the arrest of bleeding with haemostatic agents, excluding vitamin K, blood products and agents for topical use. A group of experts in the field of haemostasis and clinical pharmacology was invited, together with delegates from the manufacturers of haemostatic agents, for a critical discussion.

For each commercially available haemostatic substance a detailed report was pre-circulated by one of the invited experts who had reviewed in detail the documents available in the literature and the material submitted by the manufacturer; this document was the basis of the discussion during the symposium, and the published version reflects the common opinion of the invited experts. An opportunity was offered to the manufacturers, who delegated a representative to the symposium, to comment on this final report.[1]

In order to be considered, the documents submitted to demonstrate the clinical efficacy of haemostatic agents had to be published work and had to fulfil most of the following minimum requirements:

(1) Quantitation of the measured blood loss was required, and not merely a clinical impression of the amount of blood lost, if the document pertained to a planned but «open» clinical trial.

(2) Only double-blind trials with random allocation of the placebo and experimental drug to preselected patients were considered suitable for discussion, if the blood loss had not been quantitated in a prospective trial.

(3) Definition and appropriate selection of patients admitted to the trial: all inclusion and exclusion criteria used to select patients had to be mentioned in detail.

(4) Once included in the trial, patients could be withdrawn only on the basis of strict criteria for withdrawal which had been defined in advance.

(5) A double-blind trial had to be continued for an adequate length of time if the haemostatic agent was being assessed in the prevention of bleeding in patients with a long lasting bleeding disorder.

(6) A clear and detailed statistical analysis of the results was required.

Moreover, a clear distinction between the therapeutic and prophylactic value of the haemostatic agent had to be made and applied separately to the group of patients without any major basic disorder and those with a bleeding disorder e.g.: chronic thrombocytopenia, haemophilia, Rendu-Osler telangiectasia ...

General statements not substantiated by experimental data, even when issued by well-known authorities, were not considered a reasonable basis for discussion.

[1] Spokesmen who attended the meeting: G. ANTOINE (for Choay: Paris), P. DE NICOLA (for Ravizza: Muggiò, Milano), G. DEROUAUX (for Seresci: Bruxelles), G.L. HABERLAND (for Bayer: Wuppertal), H. KJELLMAN (for Kabi: Stockholm), G. PEPEU (for Laboratori Baldacci: Pisa), E. PHILIPP (for Bayer: Wuppertal), J.V. REED (for Delandale: Canterbury), F. SCHULTE (for Hormon-Chemie: München), K. STOCKER (for Pentapharm: Basel), F.A. SUMA (for Laboratori Baldacci: Pisa).

The following experts attended the meeting:

BENNETT B. Department of Medicine, University of Aberdeen, Foresterhill, Aberdeen AB9 2ZD.

BROZOVIĆ M. Department of Haematology, Central Middlesex Hospital, London NW10 7NS.

COLLEN D. Laboratorium Bloedstolling, Departement Medische Navorsing, Academisch Ziekenhuis, Kapucijnenvoer 35, 3000 Leuven.

DE GAETANO G. Istituto di Ricerche Farmacologiche 'Mario Negri', Via Eritrea 62, 20157 Milano.

DUKES M.N.G. Staatstoezicht op de Volksgezondheid, Dokter Reijersstraat 40 Leidschendam.

FLUTE P.J. Department of Haematology, St. George's Hospital Medical School, Blackshaw Road, Tooting, London SW17 OQT.

GAFFNEY P.T. National Institute for Biological Standards and Control, Holly Hill, Hampstead, London NW3 6RB.

GARATTINI S. Istituto di Ricerche Farmacologiche 'Mario Negri', Via Eritrea 62, 20157 Milano.

HUGUES J. Secteur d'Hématologie, Institut de Médecine, Université de Liège, Boulevard de la Constitution 66, 4000 Liège.

LECHNER K.I. Medizinische Universitätsklinik, Spitalgasse 23, 1097 Wien.

MASURE R. Laboratoire d'Hémostase, Ecole de Santé Publique, Université de Louvain, Clos Chapelle-aux-Champs 30, 1200 Bruxelles.

McNICOL G.P. Department of Medicine, University of Leeds, Leeds LS1 3EX.

NILSSON I.M. Koagulationslaboratoriet, Allmänna Sjukhuset, 214 01 Malmö.

POLLER L. Department of Haematology, Withington Hospital, Manchester M20 8LR.

PRENTICE C.R.M. University Department of Medicine, Royal Infirmary, 86 Castle Street, Glasgow G4 OSF.

ROOS J. Department Inwendige Geneeskunde, Rode Kruis Ziekenhuis, 's Gravenhage.

SHARP A.A. Gibson Laboratories, Radcliffe Infirmary, Oxford.

SIXMA J.J. Afdeling Haemostase en Thrombose, Academisch Ziekenhuis, Catharijnesingel 101, Utrecht.

VAN DE LOO J. Medizinische Universitätsklinik, Westring Münster 44.

VERMYLEN J. Laboratorium Bloedstolling, Departement Medische Navorsing, Academisch Ziekenhuis, Kapucijnenvoer 35, 3000 Leuven.

VERSTRAETE M. Laboratorium Bloedstolling, Departement Medische Navorsing, Academisch Ziekenhuis, Kapucijnenvoer 35, 3000 Leuven.

VON EICKSTEDT K.W. Bundesgesundheitsamt, Dr. Werner Vossdammstrasse 62, 1 Berlin 33.

WAUTIER J.L. Service Central d'Immuno-Hématologie, Hôpital Lariboisière, 2 rue Ambroise Paré, 75475 Paris Cedex 10.

# Acknowledgements

We would like to thank Mrs. Judith Edy for her expert help in assisting with the preparation of the manuscript and Mrs. Y. Vanhulst for secretarial help; also the Nationaal Fonds voor Wetenschappelijk Onderzoek, the University of Leuven and the Ministerie van Nationale Opvoeding en Nederlandse Cultuur, Bestuur voor Internationale Culturele Betrekkingen for a grant which made the meeting in Leuven, Belgium, possible.

# Contents

# The correction of a bleeding defect

Bleeding results from ruptured blood vessels and its spontaneous arrest is called haemostasis. Extravasation will cease if the leak (hole) is blocked, or if the intravasal pressure becomes lower than the pressure outside the bleeding vessel. In smaller vessels, vasoconstriction upstream of the bleeding point will tend to equalize the intra- and extravascular pressure and so will the opening of arterio-venous shunts in the critical area, or a fall in systemic pressure, a condition often induced by anaesthetists to limit peroperative bleeding in crucial organ areas. External pressure may increase due to packed blood e.g. in a joint; an increase in viscosity can also reduce the loss of blood.

The ability to contract when divided is not confined to the arterioles and venules. It is also possessed by smaller vessels in certain organs and is due to active contraction of filamentous structures in the endothelium, resembling myofibrils. The lumen of transected capillaries probably occludes by endothelial adhesion.

The various vascular reactions play an important role in the vessels having a muscular coat but are often not enough to result in a definite arrest of bleeding. Besides the transient vascular contraction, platelet adhesion to the damaged vascular wall and aggregation, reinforced by formation of a fibrin thrombus, are required to stop bleeding in somewhat larger vessels. Vasoconstriction in the traumatized area may be due to a direct effect on the muscle fibres or to a release of vasoactive substances from the damaged tissues or from the platelets, blood cells or plasma. In some cases a vasomotor nerve stimulation cannot be ruled out. It is indeed known that aggregated platelets liberate the vasoconstrictor 5-hydroxytryptamine and also adrenaline, noradrenaline and other vasoactive substances. In addition there are the vasoactive peptides of the bradykinin group which are activated by the Hageman factor (factor XII), the same factor which initiates the blood coagulation cascade. It thus seems that coagulation and kinin formation are two intimately connected mechanisms. Kinins are known to cause vasodilatation and increased permeability resulting in loss of plasma from the intravascular compartment and thus red-cell packing.

## The correction of a bleeding defect in patients with a lifelong bleeding disorder.

Several lifelong bleeding disorders are due to a deficiency of one or, occasionally, several coagulation factors. In most instances bleeding can be prevented or treated by intravenous transfusion of a concentrate of the missing clotting factor.

In congenital fibrinogen deficiency the initial dose is 1.0 g fibrinogen per 10 kg body weight followed by 150 mg per 10 kg body weight daily until the haemostatic level of 60 mg per 100 ml is reached. As the half-life of this protein is 4-6 days, transfusion for the control of spontaneous haemorrhages or after surgery need only be given every two and a half days. Congenital prothrombin deficiency is very rare and so are congenital factor VII or X deficiencies. Concentrates of factor II, IX and X are commercially available and some of them also contain large amounts of factor VII. The minimal level of prothrombin required for normal haemostasis is 30-40 percent and this value can also be reached by transfusion of 15-20 ml of normal plasma per kg body weight. The half-life of prothrombin is 3-4 days. A minimal level of 5-10 percent factor VII (half-life 4-6 hours), and 15-20 percent factor X (half-life 2-3 days) are required for normal haemostasis. Fibrinogen, prothrombin and factors VII and X are also stable in frozen or dried plasma. Fresh frozen plasma and, to a minor extent, cryoprecipitate can be used to treat the few patients with a congenital deficiency of factor V (half-life 12-36 hours). Factor XI deficiency is seldom a problem except where surgery is contemplated. This factor is stable in plasma (initial transfusion dose 10-20 ml/kg body weight) and has a long in vivo half-disappearance time (60 hours) so that the maintenance dose (5 ml/kg body weight) may be given every third day. Hereditary factor XIII deficiency is associated with spontaneous haemorrhagic phenomena and poor wound healing. As the concentration required for haemostasis is very low (1-2%) compared to that in normal plasma, and the half-disappearance time is long (3-4 days), fresh frozen plasma administered every third day suffices; repeated administration of just 15 ml/kg body weight at monthly intervals is enough for an effective prophylaxis. Fibrinogen concentrates are also a good source of Factor XIII.

In classical haemophilia A, the administration of 1 unit of factor VIII per kg body weight corresponds to an increase of 2% factor VIII in the plasma; the half-life of factor VIII is between 10 and 12 hours and the plasma level required to stop bleeding is 15-20%. This means that 10 units of factor VIII per kg body weight need to be given twice daily.

In the less common haemophilia B or Christmas disease, daily infusions of factor IX are usually sufficient because of its longer half-life (18-24 hours). Due to the larger body compartment space in which factor IX is distributed, 1 unit of factor IX administered per kg body weight will increase the circulating level by 1% at most; the recommended daily dose to maintain a safe circulating level of 20% is therefore at least 40 units per kg body weight.

In haemophilic patients with an inhibitor to factor VIII or IX one can try to overcome the antibody by large doses of high potency preparations of the missing coagulation factor; other methods are exchange transfusion, immunosuppressive therapy and, more recently, partially activated concentrates of factor II, (VII), IX and X.

The molecular defects in the autosomal dominant von Willebrand's disease are more complex and the bleeding manifestations often as severe as in haemophilia. Replacement therapy is best using fresh frozen plasma or cryoprecipitated factor VIII, and should preferably be started two days before an operation.


## The correction of bleeding defects in patients with an acquired haemostasis defect present before operation

Drugs affecting platelet function (e.g. aspirin, dipyridamole and congeners, sulfinpyrazone, hydroxychloroquine and intravenous dextran) may be potentially hazardous in surgical patients. A limited number of controlled clinical studies have revealed that there is a small but increased risk of surgical bleeding in patients receiving these drugs, but further studies are required to determine whether this possibly harmful effect outweighs the benefit of preventing deep venous thrombosis. In case of doubt, transfusion of fresh platelets is the only way to compensate for dysfunctioning platelets.

The most common causes of an acquired defect of blood coagulation factors are hepatic insufficiency, the non-availability of vitamin K or, less frequently, the known or hidden intake of coumarin drugs. Surgeons sometimes prescribe broad-spectrum oral antibiotics to sterilize the gut, a procedure which, of course, also suppresses the intestinal vitamin K source. There may also be a failure to absorb vitamin K from the gut, as in obstructive jaundice or steatorrhoea. When the liver function is normal, vitamin K (25-50 mg) administered intravenously will satisfactorily augment the depressed synthesis of the coagulation factors; in the presence of severe liver insufficiency vitamin K will be of no avail and fresh frozen or dried plasma or the appropriate concentrates of the missing coagulation factors will have to be given.

Uraemic patients often have a bleeding tendency with a long bleeding time mainly related to platelet dysfunction. These patients have an abnormal platelet release reaction probably due to a retained metabolite. This explains why the defect can be corrected by haemodialysis or peritoneal dialysis.

Patients with thrombocytopenia or with essential thrombocythaemia have a spontaneous bleeding tendency with skin ecchymoses, epistaxis, bleeding from the gums and gastrointestinal haemorrhage. If an operation has to be performed on a thrombocytopenic patient, platelets concentrated from fresh plasma should be administered and, as a rule of thumb, concentrates of 1 or 2 units of blood per 5 kg body weight are often recommended. The *in vivo* survival of platelet concentrates can be extremely short (1-2 hours) in thrombocytopenia due to an immunisation process.

Abnormalities of platelet function are also found in patients with multiple myeloma and macroglobulinaemia as these abnormal proteins interfere with the thrombin-fibrinogen reaction. If in addition there is an apparent decrease in factor VIII by adsorption on γA or γM globulins, *in vivo* correction may be tried by administering large doses of penicillamine or 2-mercaptoethanol, and even better is plasmapheresis which removes the excess protein and also reduces the hypovolaemia.

### The specific treatment of prolonged bleeding in patients with a normal haemostatic mechanism before operation

Prolonged bleeding in patients with pre-operatively normal haemostasis frequently occurs during operation. Bleeding can be due to errors in technique such as inadvertent injury of a major vessel or imperfect ligation, and this is often discovered on re-exploration of the wound.

Multiple individual ligations take time and each surgeon has to make a balance between the safety of surgical haemostasis and the length of the operative procedure. There are certain operations which, by nature of their dissections, are more frequently accompanied by abundant oozing, often without localizable or clampable bleeding points.

In other circumstances the area under operation may stay dry as long as the blood pressure remains at a low level (giving a false sense of security) but start to bleed once the pressure is normalized.

Certain anaesthetic procedures associated with $CO_2$ retention, hypoxia or an increased venous pressure are also associated with a greater blood loss; there is still conflicting evidence about the value of spinal anaesthesia as regards this point.

Bleeding in surgical patients can also result from errors in drug administration: an overdose of heparin, administration of a normal dose of heparin but in a highly susceptible patient (e.g. with thrombocytopenia), or an error in heparin neutralization. The potency of each batch of heparin may vary, but in general 1 mg heparin is neutralized by 1 to 1.5 mg of protamine salt. After intravenous heparin administration the quantity of protamine required for neutralization decreases progressively as the heparin effect wears off. When subcutaneous depot heparin is to be neutralized, one should remember that protamine is more rapidly metabolized than heparin (a difference of approximately 2 hours). More protamine is required for neutralization of beef lung heparin than of the same amount of hog intestinal mucosa heparin, because the former contains more non-anticoagulant substances, such as chondractin, which react with the protamine.

A haemorrhagic tendency may develop immediately after a mismatched blood transfusion, blood oozing from the cut surfaces of the incision, fresh puncture sites, gums or uterus (in postpartum cases). In an anaesthetized patient, generalized bleeding is often the first if not the cardinal sign of an incompatible blood transfusion; the appearance of haemoglobin in the urine is only discovered later. Large quantities of group O blood should not be administered. even under emergency conditions, since subsequently transfused type-specific blood will be haemolysed. Only large quantities of O, Rh-negative erythrocytes can be recommended in these circumstances. As little as 150 ml of incompatible blood can initiate haemolysis in an adult and cause widespread intravascular coagulation. The danger of further defibrination persists as long as the products of haemolysis remain in the circulation.

Generalized bleeding may occur when large volumes (more than 5 litres within 24 hours in an adult) of compatible banked blood are transfused, because stored blood is lacking in factor V and VIII activity and has a reduced number of functioning platelets. The constant bleeding may act as an indication for continued transfusion, setting up a vicious circle which can be broken only by the administration of freshly collected blood. Massive transfusion of ordinary stored blood induces a thrombocytopenic state and a low level of the labile factors V and VII by dilution of the patient's blood. Moreover the recipient's platelets may be destroyed if platelet blood group antibodies or non-specific antiplatelet factors are present in the transfused blood. To avoid this complication, one unit of fresh blood, preferably collected in siliconized containers or plastic bags in order to prolong platelet survival, should be transfused for every three units of banked blood. Citrate overdosage is rare because the liver can-metabolize 0.03-0.04 mmoles per kg per min, which allows the safe transfusion of 2 litres of citrated blood in 20 minutes; cardiac arrest is likely to preceed any interference of hypocalcaemia with haemostasis. Nevertheless some anaesthetists administer routinely 10 ml of calcium gluconate 10% per litre citrated blood when the calculated rate of transfusion is above 2 litres of blood per 20 minute period.

Epistaxis, prolonged post-traumatic haemorrhage and surgical bleeding may occur in patients who have received large infusions of plasma expanders such as dextran, gelatin or polyvinyl pyrrolidone. These materials inhibit platelet function, interfere with fibrinogen conversion and have a blood dilution effect. For this reason a dose of 2 g dextran 40 (Rheomacrodex®) or 1 g dextran 70 (Macrodex®) per kg body weight per day should not be exceeded.

Surgical haemorrhage can also be due to haemostatic imbalance induced during or after operation. The main types are diffuse vascular coagulation uncomplicated by an adequate synthesis of coagulation factors, and local or regional massive fibrin deposition (e.g. retroplacentar haematoma); both conditions are most often associated with secondary or reactive fibrinolysis.

**Treatment of bleeding without apparent surgical, haematological or other cause**

This steady loss of blood is a serious accompaniment of many surgical procedures and cases of major trauma. Surgery is inevitably accompanied by some bleeding although the surgeon strives to devise techniques which are relatively bloodless. Replacement of lost blood is at present so familiar a decision that many surgeons underrate its still possible medical complications (abscess formation, wound disruption, hepatitis) and economic implications. A direct approach to the prevention or reduction of bleeding during and after surgery consists of electrocoagulation, suture ligature, reduction of systemic blood pressure (carrying the risk of cerebral and myocardial infarction in elderly men), blockage of the sympathetic nervous system, towel application and the use of gauze packs, cooling of the irrigation fluid in certain operations, etc.

When these measures fail, when bleeding is located at sites difficult to reach, and when no technical or other causes for faulty haemostasis can be found, a drug reducing bleeding would be indicated, were such an agent available at present. Physicians and surgeons are prepared to try any systematically administered drug, even one with a slim chance of success. No doubt the numerous 'haemostatic agents' have given the relative benefit of some hope, if not a false security, in many dramatic instances, but in practice have given very little clinical benefit to the patient. Each of them has had its vogue and many have survived by means of obsolete traditions to the present time. Although many of the presently available haemostatic drugs are purported to reduce blood loss during and after surgical operations, more recent and stringent clinical trials have been unable to confirm this clinical property. Perhaps no other single mode of therapy is applied with such empiricism and so illogically as the administration of systemic haemostatic drugs. Critical re-evaluation of these drugs is therefore a timely exercise.

# Report on a tissue extract[1]: Clauden®

## Chemical definition of the drug

A tissue extract prepared from fresh? animal tissues. No other data are available.

## Theoretical mode of action

Accelerates coagulation *in vitro* and *in vivo* by enhancing prothrombin conversion to thrombin.

*In vitro* the addition of Clauden® shortens the whole blood clotting time, recalcification time (with and without heparin), one-stage and two-stage prothrombin time, but has little effect on the thrombin time (Egger 1954). The efficacy of coagulation is improved as judged by the prothrombin consumption test and thromboelastograph tracings (Egger 1954).

*In vivo* the effect of intravenously injected Clauden® lasts for 1 hour showing a maximum effect at 30-45 minutes. Whole blood clotting time, recalcification time, and one- and two-stage prothrombin times are shortened (Egger, 1954). Thromboplastin generation is accelerated and the activation plateau is reached earlier than before injection (Kommerell, 1960). The addition of platelets does not alter the effect of Clauden® *in vitro*. Haiböck (1972) performed the one-stage prothrombin time, bleeding time and whole blood clotting time on 15 healthy individuals and 15 surgical patients after the injection of Clauden®, and showed a shortening in all tests. The results are summarized in Table 1.

---

1. Other tissue extracts: Coagulen®, Coazimol®, Frénovex®, Hemostatique Ercé®, Manetol®, Thrombocytine®.

*Table 1.* Effect of Clauden ® on clotting tests (data of Haiböck)

| Test | % Shortening | |
|------|:---:|:---:|
| | patients | healthy subjects |
| one-stage prothrombin time | 7.9 | 5.0 |
| bleeding time | 25.0 | 12.0 |
| whole blood clotting time | 24.5 | 8.0 |

## Animal and human pharmacology

No systematic studies are available. It is claimed that Clauden® is equally effective when administered orally, by inhalation, or by subcutaneous, intramuscular or intravenous injection. After intravenous injection, the effect on blood coagulation is immediate, reaches a maximum at 30-45 minutes and lasts for at least 1 hour.

## Clinical efficacy

Numerous reports on the effects of Clauden® in individual patients or small groups of patients exist in the German and Japanese literature between 1918 and 1942. A summary of the more recent data is given in Table 2.

*Table 2.* Subjects given Clauden ® i.v.

| Subjects | No. | Author | Year | Effect |
|----------|-----|--------|------|--------|
| Healthy | 11 | Egger | 1954 | Shortening of clotting times for up to 60 min. |
| Healthy | 20 | Kommerell | 1960 | Acceleration of thromboplastin generation 15 to 60 min after injection. |
| Healthy | 15 | Haiböck | 1972 | Little effect on clotting tests* 15 min after injection. |
| Surgical patients | 15 | Haiböck | 1972 | Shortening of clotting tests* 15 min after injection. |

* See Table 1.

## Side effects

None reported after a single 50 ml dose i.v. in 5 healthy individuals (Kommerell 1960) or 80-90 ml i.v. daily in several patients (Cioran, 1935). No evidence of disseminated intravascular clotting was found on autopsy in patients who had been given large doses of Clauden® before death (Kelch 1927).

## Recommended dose

Intravenous injection: 10-20 ml 2-3 times daily. Intramuscular injection: 10 ml 2-3 times daily. Orally: 2 tablets 3 times daily.

## Conclusions

This tissue extract of unknown chemical composition probably enhances prothrombin conversion to thrombin via 'thromboplastin-like' action, and causes shortening of coagulation times *in vivo* and *in vitro*. Pharmacological data and clinical trials are not available.

REFERENCES

CIORAN (1935) *Wien. med. Wschr.* 38. Quoted in manufacturer's information.
EGGER E. (1954) Experimentelle Untersuchungen über die Wirkung von Clauden. *Arzneimittel-Forsch.* 11, 657.
HAIBOCK H. F. (1972) Clinical and experimental investigations of a physiological haemostatic agent. *Z. Ther.* 6, 339.
KELCH (1927) *Med. Klin.* 40. Quoted in manufacturer's information.
KOMMERELL B. (1960) The coagulation activation effect of Clauden as established by the Thrombokinase formation test. *Münch. med. Wschr.* 102, 1332.

# Report on a preparation of phospholipids: Tachostyptan®

## Chemistry

According to the chromatographic studies of Deutsch and Fischer (1963), Tachostyptan® is a micellar suspension of the following phospholipids: phosphatidylcholine, phosphatidylserine, phosphatidylethanolamine, phosphatidylinositol, lysolethicin and lysocephalin. Their quantitative relationship is unknown. It contains at least eleven amino acids and traces of peptides but no protein. The substance is manufactured from fresh animal brain (presumably bovine and porcine), is stable at $+4°C$ for several years, unstable at $-20°C$ or if otherwise frozen, and also unstable at room temperature or in contact with air.

## Experimental coagulation studies

**In vitro.** Several investigators have independently shown that dilutions of Tachostyptan® shorten the partial thromboplastin time (Deutsch and Fischer 1963, Mitrenga 1972), the RVV coagulation time (Deutsch and Fischer 1963), the thromboplastin generation test according to Biggs and Douglas (Deutsch and Fischer 1963, Zürn 1956), the recalcification time (Deutsch, 1952; Mitrenga, 1972), the thrombin time (Deutsch, 1952; Mitrenga, 1972), and the r and k values of the thromboelastogram (Herrmann, 1955).

The different authors agree that this is true for concentrations between $6.6 \times 10^{-2}$ mg/ml and $6.6 \times 10^{-4}$ mg/ml, with a maximum activity between $3.3 \times 10^{-2}$ and $6.6 \times 10^{-3}$ mg/ml. High concentrations such as those present in the original preparation (2 mg phospholipids/ml) exert a slight inhibitory effect on coagulation.

The accelerating activity of diluted Tachostyptan® was comparable to that of alcohol ether extracts of human platelets (platelet factor 3) or of human brain tissue. Deutsch and Fischer (1963) therefore proposed replacing these latter reagents by Tachostyptan® in the following test procedures: partial thromboplastin time, thromboplastin generation test and determination of factor X. For this purpose the manufacturer has provided a specially purified preparation for laboratory use, called 'Tachostyptest®'.

**In vivo.** Deutsch (1952) described a marked shortening of the clotting time, recalcification time, bleeding time of Duke, and the k value of the thromboelastogram in normal volunteers following an injection of Tachostyptan®. Similar results have been published by Schimpf *et al.* (1972) who measured prothrombin consumption and thrombin generation. Pohlreich's experiment on endotoxin-induced shock reactions in rabbits revealed a significant enhancement of these reactions (fibrin deposits in lung, liver and kidney and decrease of coagulation factors) by Tachostyptan®.

## Pharmacokinetics, toxicity

No published pharmacokinetic studies in animals or humans are available. Deutsch (1952) reported no shock or other allergic reaction in guinea pigs when successive injections of Tachostyptan® were administered within a 20-day period. According to Reichel *et al.* (1953), no adverse reactions of circulatory or cardiac function could be observed in normal human subjects following slow i.v. injection of 10 ml Tachostyptan®. Fast injection may decrease the blood pressure.

## Clinical studies

No controlled clinical trials on the haemostatic effect of Tachostyptan® in any clinical condition are available. Numerous case reports, however, claim a beneficial effect in the various conditions for which the drug is recommended by the manufacturer. Some of them should be mentioned. Schimpf *et al.* (1972) were able to demonstrate, in 12 uraemic patients, that the i.v. infusion of 10 ml Tachostyptan® normalized the pathological thrombin generation and prothrombin consumption for 3 hours. Similar effects have been described by Beck (1968). In dentistry good postoperative haemostasis was described in patients with prolonged bleeding and/or clotting times (Herrmann, 1955) and in von Willebrand patients undergoing tooth extraction (Utz, 1968). The experience in thrombopenic or thrombopathic patients is controversial (Marx, 1967).

## Recommended dosage

According to the manufacturer and to most of the authors, slow intravenous injection or infusion of 10 ml Tachostyptan® provides an optimal effect for 3 hours. Vials of 5 ml and 10 ml, containing 2 mg phospholipids/ml, are available.

## Conclusions

Tachostyptan® – a phospholipid preparation from animal brain tissue – accelerates blood clotting *in vitro* as well as *in vivo*. Controlled clinical trials on its effect as a haemostatic agent are not available. The substance is well tolerated. It seems worthwhile to study its haemostatic effect, especially in patients with uraemic or thrombopenic haemorrhagic diatheses.

REFERENCES

BECK I. (1968) *Untersuchungen über die Verminderung der Thrombinbildung bei chronischer und akuter Niereninsuffizienz und ihrer Ursachen.* Thesis, School of Medicine, Munich.
DEUTSCH E. (1952) Der Wirkungsmechanismus von 'Hämostyptikum Schoch'. *Arzneimittel-Forsch.* 2, 470.
DEUTSCH E. and FISCHER M. (1963) Die Verwendung eines stabilen Phospholipidpräparates als Thrombozytenersatz bei Gerinnungsanalysen. *Arzneimittel-Forsch.* 13, 439.
HERRMANN H. (1955) Die Behandlung van Blutungen mit Organextrakten (Tachostyptan). *Dtsch. zahnärztl. Z.* 10, 1313.
MARX R. (1967) Behandlung von Thrombozytopenien. *Therapiewoche* 17, 737.
MITRENGA D. (1972) *In vitro-Untersuchungen parenteral anwendbarer Hämostyptika.* Thesis, School of Medicine, Cologne.
POHLREICH H. (1971) *Blutgerinnung und Histologie nach sukzessiver intravenöser Injektion von Endotoxin und gerinnungsaktivem phospholipoidhaltigem Hirnextrakt bei Kaninchen.* Thesis, School of Medicine, Heidelberg.
REICHEL H.H., MARTINI F. and BLEICHERT A. (1953) Untersuchungen über die Kreislaufwirkung eines neuen Haemostypticums. *Arzneimittel-Forsch.* 3, 252.
SCHIMPF K., HANF-HOPPE H.W. and IMMICH H. (1972) Intravenous infusion of a standardised coagulation active phospholipid complex in uremic coagulation deficiency. *Thrombos. Diathes. haemorrh. (Stuttg.)* 27, 554.

Utz W. (1968) Über die zahnärztlich-chirurgische Behandlung von Patienten mit v. Willebrand-Jürgensscher Erkrankung. *Dtsch. zahnärztl. Z.* 23, 464.

Zurn H. (1956) Untersuchungen zur Gerinnungsaktivität verschiedener Schlangengifte und des Tachostyptan als Beitrag zur Physiologie der Thrombokinasebildung. *Folia haemat. (Lpz.)* 74, 402.

# Comments by the manufacturer of Tachostyptan®

**by F. Schulte, Hormon-Chemie, München**

(1) Tachostyptan® is a procoagulative haemostatic. Its phospholipid composition and its physiological effect (*in vitro* as well as *in vivo*) have been well analysed and proved to be analogous to that of platelet factor 3 (Deutsch and Fischer, 1963; Egli, 1961; Fischer, 1964; Mitrenga, 1972; Pohlreich, 1971; Schimpf *et al.*, 1972; Zürn, 1956). Thus the procoagulative activity of a 1:50 dilution is equal to a suspension of 300,000 thrombocytes per mm$^3$ (Egli, 1961).

(2) The importance of the procoagulative phospholipids for an adequate thrombin formation on the one hand (Fig. 1) and the importance of a sufficient thrombin formation for complete haemostasis on the other hand illustrate clearly and in the best way the theoretical mode of action as a haemostatic agent and the therapeutic concept of Tachostyptan.

(3) The quantitative relationship of the procoagulative phospholipids (lipid thromboplastin according to Hecht) of Tachostyptan® has not yet been completely investigated. Irrespective of this, the procoagulative activity of lipid thromboplastin depends, as is known, not only on the qualitative and quantitative chemical composition of its single phospholipid molecules but especially on the physicochemical properties of the superstructure of the phospholipid micelles composed of these molecules.
A similar situation exists e.g. in the case of heparin or antihaemophilic globulin. Preparations of both these substances have no exact chemical definitions but have been defined with regard to their biological activity. The procoagulative activity of each batch of Tachostyptan® is standardized by means of a quantitative one-stage method for determining platelet factor 3 (Egli, 1961).

(4) A dose of 10 ml of Tachostyptan® not only affects patients with a defect or insufficient platelet factor 3 (normalization of the prothrombin

*Fig. 1.* Scheme of blood coagulation (partly according to E.F. Mammen)

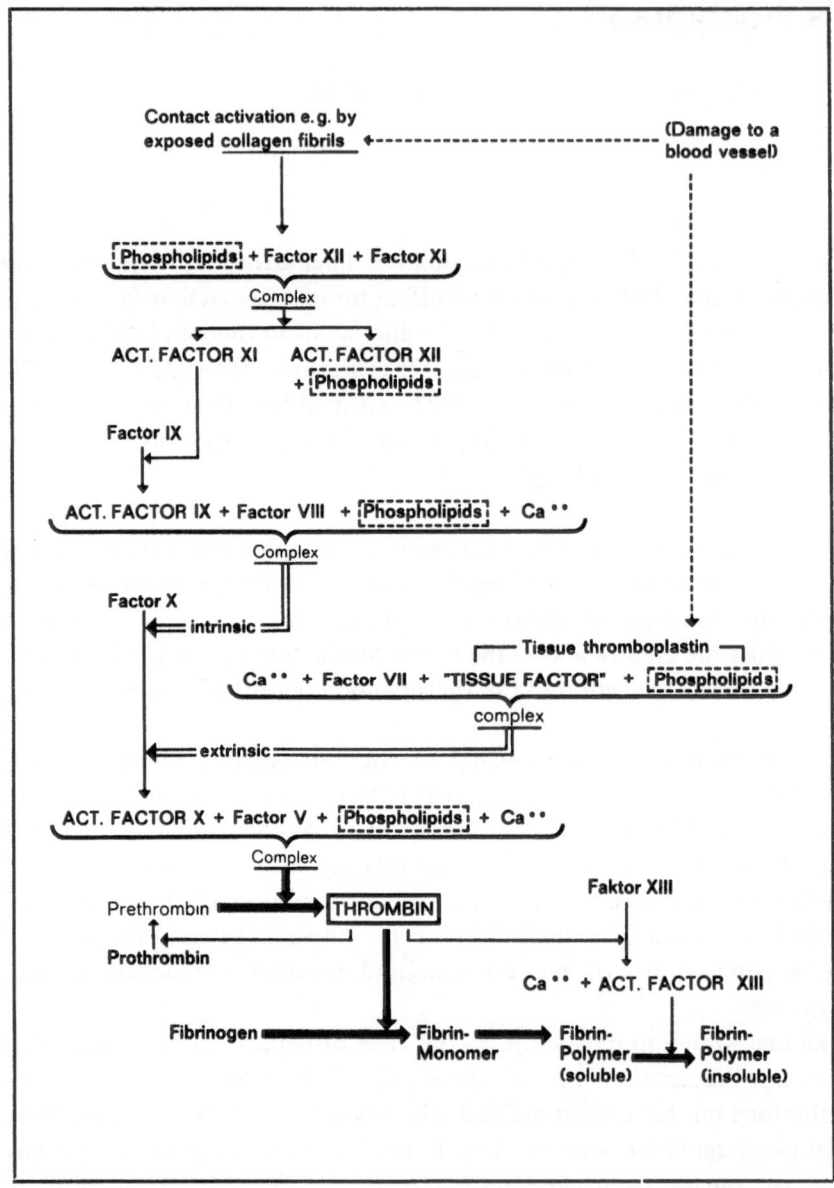

consumption test and the thrombin generation test), but also produces a statistically significant increase in the prothrombin consumption and the thrombin generation in healthy control persons (Schimpf *et al.*, 1972).

(5) By means of this increased generation of thrombin and consumption of prothrombin, the effect of an infusion of 10 ml of Tachostyptan® is measurable for 3 hours, whereas the effect of 10 ml of injected Tachostyptan® only lasts for $1^1/_2$ hours (Schimpf et al., 1972). This, and the fact that a single dose of Tachostyptan® given 2 hours before an injection of endotoxin still slightly enhances the degree of the produced disseminated intravascular coagulation (DIC) in rabbits (Pohlreich, 1971), give some preliminary pharmacokinetic indications.

(6) It is possible to conclude from 5) that a haemostyptic therapy with a substitute of platelet factor 3 has a good applicability. Of course – as must be expected from a true procoagulative agent – the application of Tachostyptan® is contraindicated in cases of DIC.
If required the haemostyptic therapy with Tachostyptan®, or rather its procoagulative effect, can be controlled by the antithrombin effect of a dose of heparin.

(7) Since its introduction, Tachostyptan® has been administered clinically as a procoagulative agent in millions of cases. In more than 1000 cases clinical trials have shown Tachostyptan® to be a real haemostatic. New and controlled clinical trials on the haemostatic effect and on the clinical efficacy of Tachostyptan® are underway.

REFERENCES

DEUTSCH E. and FISCHER M. (1963) Die Verwendung eines stabilen Phospholipidpräparates als Thrombozytenersatz bei Gerinnungsanalysen. *Arzneimittel-Forsch.* 13, 439.
EGLI H. (1961) Eine quantitative Einstufenmethode zur Bestimmung des Thrombozyten faktors 3. *Thrombos. Diathes. haemorrh. (Stuttg.)* 6, 533.
FISCHER M. (1964) Ein stabiles Phospholipidreagens als Thrombozytenersatz bei Gerinnungsanalysen. *Arzneimittel-Forsch.* 14, 1321.
MITRENGA D. (1972) *In vitro-Untersuchungen parenteral anwendbarer Hämostyptika.* Thesis, School of Medicine, Cologne.
POHLREICH H. (1971) *Blutgerinnung und Histologie nach sukzessiver intravenöser Injektion von Endotoxin und gerinnungsaktivem phospholipoidhaltigem Hirnextrakt bei Kaninchen.* Thesis, School of Medicine, Heidelberg.
SCHIMPF K., HANF-HOPPE H.W. and IMMICH H. (1972) Intravenous infusion of a standardised coagulation active phospholipid complex in uremic coagulation deficiency. *Thrombos. Diathes. haemorrh. (Stuutg.)* 27, 554.
ZURN H. (1956) Untersuchungen zur Gerinnungsaktivität verschiedener Schlangengifte und des Tachostyptan als Beitrag zur Physiologie der Thrombokinasebildung. *Folia haemat. (Lpz.)* 74, 402.

# Report on a preparation of oxalic and malonic acids: Koagamin®

Koagamin® is an aqueous acid solution of oxalic and malonic acids given by intravenous or intramuscular injection in a dosage of 2 and 3 ml respectively. In 1939 Steinberg and Brown claimed that oxalic acid accelerated the coagulation time. Steinberg and Brown in 1939 described beneficial effects in patients suffering from various defects of haemostasis. Herbst and Weinstein (1944) claimed acceleration of the bleeding time and of the capillary tube clotting time in normals and operative patients although none were grossly abnormal initially.

The drug has apparently been discontinued.

REFERENCES

STEINBERG A. and BROWN W.R. (1939) A new concept regarding the mechanism of clotting and the control of haemorrhage. *Amer. J. Physiol.* 126, 638.
HERBST W.P. and WEINSTEIN J.J. (1944) Observations on the action of Koagamin. *J. Urol. (Baltimore)* 51, 325.

# Report on a preparation of butyl alcohol: Haemostypticum Revici®

## Chemical definition

Haemostypticum Revici® (HR) is simply butanol (butyl alcohol). The preparation is named after its initiator, Dr. E. Revici, director of the Institute of Applied Biology in New York. HR contains n-butanol, citric acid and disaccharides. According to Kuschinsky (1968) the preparation sometimes contained trillium, a chemically undefined substance (*Trillium* is a genus of liliaceous plants) which is also supposed to have haemostyptic activity. HR is marketed in capsules in an oral mixture and as injections in saline.

## Theoretical mode of action

Dr. Revici postulated that bleeding occurs at places of local alkalosis in injured or diseased tissues. He thought that butanol could change this local alkalosis without influencing the clotting system or bleeding time. It seems uncertain whether the alcohol or the citric acid is the active substance in this postulate. The quantity of citric acid (2.5 mg/5 ml), however, would seem to be insufficient to produce any physiological effect. In our opinion a well-performed bleeding time should demostrate such a local influence.

## Pharmacology and toxicology

Starting from his theory of local alkalosis, Dr. Revici measured pH values in experimentally-induced bleeding skin defects in 164 rats. 24 hours after the wound was made, the local pH had risen from 7.30 to 7.72. Afterwards it fell to 7.60 in 48 hours and to 7.32 in 72 hours. In contrast to ethanol and propanol, butanol showed an acidifying influence. We were not able to find exact figures on this statement.

In the pharmacological department in Mainz (Kuschinsky *et al.*, 1968), investigations were performed on the bleeding time in the ears of rabbits. The bleeding time according to Roskam was measured in a control group of 15 rabbits, in 14 rabbits which had received a standard dose of 0.28 ml HR per 2 kg body weight intravenously, in 6 rabbits which had received a 10-fold dose at the same time (1 minute post-traumatically) and in some rabbits (no exact figure) which received the intravenous injection 1.5 minutes before the determination of the bleeding time. No statistically significant difference was observed (Table 1).

*Table 1.* KUSCHINSKY G., LANG M. and WOLLERT H. (1968) Untersuchungen über die Wirkung von Butanol als Haemostypticum. *Dtsch. med. Wschr.* 93, 1443.

| n | Haemostypticum Revici | Bleeding time | | p (versus controls) |
|---|---|---|---|---|
| 15 | controls | 281.3 s ± 11.5 | | |
| 14 | 0.28 ml/2 kg i.v. | 309.3 | 23.4 | <0.05 |
| 6 | 10 x 0.28 ml/2 kg | 266.7 | 10.7 | 0.025>p>0.01 |
| ? | preventive intravenous injection of 0.28 ml/2 kg | 309.3 | 23.4 | |
| | gastric tube | | | |
| 16 | controls | 373.4 | 22.7 | |
| 15 | 0.28 ml/2 kg | 404.0 | 36.9 | 0.01>p>0.05 |

Orally given doses had no effect on either the bleeding time or the blood pressure in rats. The introduction of a gastric tube prolonged the bleeding time by a hundred seconds.

Poliwoda and Deinhardt (1973) examined the bleeding time in rats at the request of the manufacturer. They provoked a bleeding from mesenteric vessels injured by laser rays. The results, which were not published as far as we know, are summarized in a letter to the manufacturer. Rats showed a bleeding time of 33 s, and, 5 min after a standard dose of HR, 23 s; the spread in this test, however, is high. (Table 2).

*Table 2.* POLIWODA H. and DEINHARDT J. (1973) Bleeding time in mesenterial vessels of rats, injured by laser ray. Personal letter.

| n | | bleeding time | | p |
|---|---|---|---|---|
| 191 | controls | 33.35 s | ± 22.5 | < 0.0005 |
| 191 | 5 min after Haemostypticum Revici | 23.3 s | ± 17.6 | |

**Clinical results**

*In patients with bleeding disorders.* No data are available.

*In patients without bleeding disorders.* The manufacturer recommends the use of HR in bleeding episodes after operations on the prostate, the uterus and the gall-bladder, after tonsillectomy, in cases of retinal haemorrhage and after tooth extraction.

Scher (1964) gave HR to 3200 patients undergoing plastic surgery of the nose. He saw no bleeding on the 7th postoperative day except in 12 patients who had refused the administration; 10 ml HR i.v. subsequently stopped the bleeding even in these patients.

Ravich (1949) used HR after prostatectomy: 4% of patients receiving HR needed a blood transfusion, whereas 20% of those who did not receive the drug required a transfusion.

In general practice Maier-Bosse saw a beneficial influence of HR in cancer, nephrolithiasis, retinitis diabetica, hypermenorrhoea and accidents. Gins (1962) had success in dentistry, and Faber and Merz (1967) in veterinary practice.

Stieve (1962) saw haemostyptic activity in patients with haemorrhagic gastritis whereas he failed to observe thromboembolic phenomena after administration of HR.

**Side effects**

14 unpublished studies were performed in the Laboratory for Pharmacology and Toxicology in Hamburg (Leuschner 1974, 1975) on dogs, mice, rats, pregnant rabbits and pregnant rats. The i.v. $LD_{50}$ was 7.9 ml per kg. There were no signs of fetal malformations. Local or systemic

allergic reactions after i.v. or i.a. injections were not observed. Haemolysis *in vitro* did not occur after adding a therapeutic dose.


## Recommended dose

Capsules: therapeutic or prophylactic, 3 capsules
Oral liquid 1-2 ampoules of 20 ml
Intravenous injection: 5-10 ml slowly.


## Conclusions

Few pharmacological and toxicological data are available on HR; clinical information is scarce and open to criticism. The theoretical basis for the activity of HR is gravely undermined by Kuschinsky's examinations. There are no double-blind prospective trials on series of randomized groups of patients.
On the basis of the available information we conclude that the haemostyptic activity of HR is entirely speculative.

REFERENCES

FABER VON T. and MERZ O. (1967) Haemostypticum-Revici in der Veterinärmedizin. *Prakt. Tierarzt* 48, 3.
GINS H. (1962) Neuartige und zuverlässige Blutstillung auf oralem Wege durch 'Haemostypticum-Revici'. *Zahnärztl. Rdsch.* 71, 4.
KUSCHINSKY G., LANG M. and WOLLERT U. (1968) Untersuchungen über die Wirkungen von Butanol als Hämostypticum. *Dtsch. med. Wschr.* 93, 1443.
LEUSCHNER F. (1974, 1975) Letters to manufacturer.
MAIER-BOSSE D. (1962) Ein neues Blutstillungsmittel, Haemostypticum-Revici. *Landarzt* 38, 1052.
POLIWODA H. and DEINHARDT J. (1973) Letter to manufacturer.
RAVICH R.A. and RAVICH A. (1949) *J. Urol.* (Baltimore) 62, 629.
REVICI E. (1961) *Research in Physiopathology as Basis of Guided Chemotherapy,* Princeton N.J.
REVICI E. (1965) *Die Pharmakologie und Toxikologie des n-Butanol.* New York.
REVICI E., HUESCA-MEJA C. and RAVICH R.A. (1949) *Bull. Inst. Appl. Biol.* 1, 73.
SCHER S.L. (1964) Eine neue Methode zur Behandlung und Prophylaxe von Blutungen, beobachtet bei mehr als 3200 Fällen. *Chirurg* 35, 435.
SCHWARZHAUPT K.G. CHEM. FABRIK KOLN. Prospectus to 'Haemostypticum Revici'.
STIEVE R. (1962) Beobachtungen über Blutstillung bei parenchymatösen Blutungen. *Landarzt* 38, 796.

# Report on sodium 4-aminonaphthalene-1-sulphonate: Naphthionin®

## Chemical definition

Naphthionin® is sodium 4-aminonaphthalene-1-sulphonate.

This substance is related to Congo Red which had been claimed, in 1933, to be of value in the treatment of the haemorrhagic tendency in thrombocytopenic purpura (Brühl, 1933).

## Theoretical mode of action as a haemostatic agent

The manner in which Naphthionin® was believed to exert its haemostatic action was by lowering the iso-electric point of fibrinogen with the result that at a pH in the region of 7.3, blood passes more easily from a sol to a gel state which facilitates haemostasis. This gel formation is possibly the reason for the perhaps spurious observations on shortening of the clotting time made with capillary tube and glass slide methods.

## Animal and human pharmacology: pharmacodynamics, pharmacokinetics, toxicology

A number of claims were made in the early 1950's that this substance had haemostatic properties in a variety of clinical situations and was reported to produce a significant shortening of the blood clotting time in man (Dubois-Ferriere, 1950). None of the clinical studies was double-blind and none, in fact, was adequately controlled. The observations on clotting times were based on observations on capillary tube or glass slide clotting tests. There was a transient but significant reduction of the bleeding time which was maximum one hour after intravenous injection but after two hours the effect had disappeared (Poller, 1955).

## Clinical efficacy in patients with a bleeding disorder

A good response was achieved in three patients suffering from severe haemorrhage who had thrombocytopenia and a platelet count under 50,000/ml (Poller and More, 1964).

## Clinical efficacy in individuals without a bleeding disorder

The effect of the intravenous administration of Naphthionin® was observed in 10 healthy young adult males (Poller, 1955). Before injection, the bleeding time, clotting time (by the Lee and White method), prothrombin time, and the heparin retarded clotting time were estimated. Ten millilitres (1 g) of the drug was injected. Bleeding, clotting, and prothrombin times were repeatedly tested at 30-minute intervals over a three-hour period while heparin-retarded tests were repeated hourly. The effect on bleeding, clotting, and prothrombin times was observed.

The significant result was the appreciable reduction of the bleeding time, which appeared to be greatest one hour after injection. The bleeding time is a crude test, yet the differences noted were marked.

In seven patients with platelet counts less than 50,000/ml but no overt haemorrhage, a significant reduction of bleeding time was obtained after the administration of Naphthionin®. In one patient with acute myeloblastic leukaemia, without overt bleeding, there was an associated defibrination but Naphthionin® produced no measurable effect on the bleeding time until fibrinogen was infused (Poller and More, 1964).

## Side effects

None reported.

## Recommended dose

1 g (10 ml) intravenously or intramuscularly followed by 0.5 − 1 g every 6 hours.

The drug is no longer available commercially.

REFERENCES

BRUHL H. (1933) Beitrage zum Krankenheitsbild and zur Behandlung des Morbus Maculosus. *Z. Kinderheilk.* 54, 159.
DUBOIS-FERRIERE H. (1950) Etude experimentale d'un nouvel hémostatique alpha-naphthionine-4-sulphonate de sodium. *Schweiz. med. Wschr.* 80, 861.
POLLER L. (1955) A study of Naphthionin, a new haemostatic drug. *J. clin. Path.* 8, 331.
POLLER L. and MORE J.R.S. (1964) A study of Naphthionin in the management of the bleeding defect in patients with thrombocytopenia. *J. clin. Path.* 17, 680.

# Report on ethamsylate[1]

## Chemical definition of ethamsylate

Ethamsylate (also known as cyclonamine) is diethylamine 2,5-dihydroxybenzenesulphonate; its structural formula is shown below:

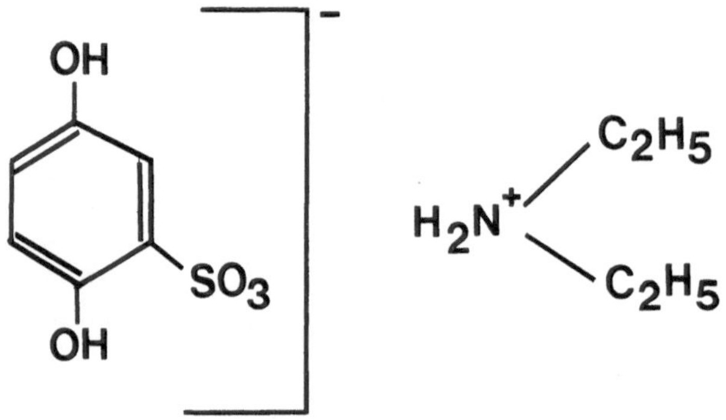

It is a white, crystalline substance, odourless, with a slight salty taste, readily soluble in water to produce a solution of pH 6.5. It is presented for clinical use in tablet form for oral administration, and in ampoules containing a solution for parenteral use.

## Theoretical mode of action of ethamsylate as a haemostatic agent

Animal experiments and clinical studies have suggested that ethamsylate increases platelet adhesiveness (or retention) to glass beads, increases capillary wall resistance and reduces the bleeding time. Ethamsylate reduces the bleeding time of both normal individuals and patients affected by various haemorrhagic conditions such as thrombocytopenia,

1. Dicynene®, Dicynone®, Mediaven®, OM-Dicinoma®.

Rendu-Osler syndrome, leukaemias (Canal, 1964; Louis and Paulus, 1967; Cajozzo *et al.*, 1973). Its effect seems to be independent of the initial value of the bleeding time or the number of platelets (Louis and Paulus, 1967).

An elegant and well conducted experimental study has demonstrated that ethamsylate is effective in reducing blood loss from a standard wound produced in pigs by means of an electric dermatome. Under the experimental conditions used, the magnitude of the reduction of bleeding was directly proportional to the severity of the unmodified bleeding (Deacock and Birley, 1969).

Using a «capillarodynamometer» in double-blind studies some authors have shown an increased capillary wall resistance in normal subjects or in patients with a haemorrhagic diathesis (liver cirrhosis, thrombocytopenia, diabetes mellitus, etc.) when ethamsylate was given (Raby and Coupier, 1965; Louis and Paulus, 1967; Prato and Fiorina, 1968; Daubresse, 1971; Cajozzo *et al.*, 1973).

An increase in platelet adhesiveness to glass following ethamsylate administration has been reported in normal individuals and in some patients with thrombocytopenia, Glanzmann thrombasthenia, von Willebrand's disease or liver cirrhosis (Migne *et al.*, 1967; Prato and Fiorina, 1968; Cagianelli *et al.*, 1968; Bizzi *et al.*, 1970).

A slight but statistically significant reduction in venous but not in capillary blood platelet count has been observed by Bizzi *et al.* (1970) in both normal and thrombocytopenic subjects one hour after i.v. administration of ethamsylate (500 mg). However, other investigators have reported no changes in venous platelet count in man or in pigs (Prato and Fiorina, 1968; Cagianelli *et al.*, 1968; Deacock and Birley, 1969). A recent report has shown that two of three rabbits which were given ethamsylate (10 mg/kg body weight, orally, for 3 consecutive days) retained normal platelet counts and platelet aggregation function after induction of the generalized Sanarelli-Schwartzman reaction with Liquoid® (Medd *et al.*, 1976).

Thrombin-induced fibrin clot retraction, thromboelastogram and plasma clotting factors are not modified by ethamsylate either in *in vitro* systems or after i.v. administration to normals or to thrombocytopenic patients (Raby and Coupier, 1965; Bizzi *et al.*, 1970). An intriguing observation, however, is that ethamsylate favours the plasma clotting process occurring at room temperature (not at 37°C) (Raby and Coupier, 1965). No effect of the drug on either pulse rate or blood pressure was observed in pigs (Deacock and Birley, 1969). In guinea pigs, ethamsylate was found to inhibit the histamine-induced papule test although it is not a general anti-histaminic substance. It is devoid of adrenergic and vasoconstrictive activity (Huguet *et al.*, 1969). In contrast, it appeared to be associated with a marked anti-hyaluronidase activity, which might help to prevent the breakdown of mucopolysaccharides in the ground substance of the capillary wall (Huguet *et al.*, 1969).

No published data are available on the pharmacokinetics of ethamsylate either in experimental animals or in man. Ethamsylate is known to remain in the blood stream as an ionized solution. There appears to be no binding to protein or the blood platelets or red cells. After i.v. injection it is rapidly absorbed into all organs (and the fetus) except the brain. It is excreted unchanged in the urine (66 to 94 percent of the administered dose within 12 hours), whereas faecal elimination is very slight. No correlation could be established between the pharmacological action of the product and its plasma levels. These data, available as a manuscript (Guidicelli, 1969), have been obtained using radioactive [$^{14}$C] ethamsy-late; they suffer, therefore from the limitations inherent in this kind of study.

## Clinical efficacy in patients with a bleeding disorder

*Renal insufficiency.* Cocconi (1968) has reported five cases of patients with renal insufficiency undergoing peritoneal dialysis; ethamsylate (500 mg i.m. or i.v.) markedly reduced the amount of haemoglobin measured in the dialysis fluid coming from the peritoneum. Haemoglobin loss was determined several times in each patient both before and after administration of the drug. It is regrettable that such an interesting observation has not been reported and analysed in greater detail.

*Menorrhagia.* Three well conducted clinical trials are available on the effect of ethamsylate in the control of menorrhagia.

In a pilot study in general practice (Jaffé and Wickham, 1973) using a double-blind cross-over technique, 26 patients with heavy menstrual bleeding were treated with ethamsylate (250 mg tablets, six times a day) or identical placebo tablets during four consecutive periods. Patients were randomly allocated to receive either ethamsylate or placebo treatment first. No other treatment for menorrhagia was given during the trial. The number of tampons used and the number of days (recorded to the nearest full day) of menstrual loss was recorded. A significant reduction (p<0.005) was found in the number of tampons per menstrual period used during ethamsylate treatment (12.7 ± 0.6) as compared to the placebo (15.9 ± 0.6).

The duration of menstrual bleeding was reduced from 5.2 ±0.1 days (placebo) to 4.8 ± 0.1 days (ethamsylate), a difference which is significant at the 5% level. The subjective assessment of the severity of bleeding also indicated the superiority of ethamsylate over placebo. No side effects were noted. No patient was withdrawn from the study. The authors stated that the trial was being continued to include a total of 50 patients.

The inclusion and exclusion criteria used to select the patients for the trial were not mentioned in detail. No evidence was provided to show that the order of treatment did not affect the reduction in blood loss. In addition, although the favourable subjective results lend weight to the significant objective results, the clinical relevance of the degree of reduction in tampon usage and of the curtailing of the period of menstrual flow observed during ethamsylate treatment is questionable. Nevertheless, the results of this pilot study point to the value of ethamsylate as an effective agent for the control of menorrhagia. This suggestion is strongly supported by the results of the second study (Campbell and Harrison, 1976). Eighteen patients complaining of primary menorrhagia and 13 patients presenting with post-intrauterine-device (IUD) menorrhagia entered this double-blind cross-over trial. Eight patients (none with an IUD) dropped out of the trial before analyzable measurements were obtained: 2 were on placebo, 2 on ethamsylate and 4 had not yet received any treatment. One additional patient was excluded from the trial since she received magnesium trisilicate, a concomitant treatment which could have affected the fate of ethamsylate. The final analysis of the results did not include this patient. Nine patients with primary menorrhagia and 13 patients with IUD menorrhagia completed the trial.

The criteria for inclusion and exclusion of patients were clearly defined. Menstrual blood losses were calculated from the results of estimations of the iron content of pads and tampons, using the appropriate haemoglobin value for each patient. Each patient was followed during one «pretrial» period and four trial periods, when she received ethamsylate (two 250 mg tablets four times a day, starting five days before the anticipated onset of menstruation and continuing for ten days) for two periods and a placebo for two periods. The allocation to ethamsylate or the placebo first was made using randomization tables.

Ethamsylate reduced the blood loss for primary menorrhagia from 126.0 ml/menstrual period (placebo treatment) to 66.6 ml (p<0.01).

Such a reduction seems to be of clinical relevance since, when menstrual blood loss exceeds 80 ml per period there is a risk of anaemia due to excessive loss of iron (Jacobs and Butler, 1965).

In the IUD menorrhagia group the mean menstrual blood loss of 64.6 ml was much lower than that in the primary menorrhagia group. With ethamsylate, blood loss was reduced to 53.5 ml/period, a decrease which, although not as striking as in the primary menorrhagia group, was still significant at the 5% level.

Since, in up to 14% of patients with an IUD, the device has to be removed because of excessive bleeding (Orlans, 1973), the favourable effect of ethamsylate observed in this trial could have some clinical relevance. Evidence was obtained that the reduction in blood loss following the use of ethamsylate was directly proportional to the blood loss during placebo, at least for blood losses above 40 ml. The order of treatment did not significantly affect the reduction in blood loss observed during ethamsylate treatment. There was insufficient evidence to prove a change in the number of tampons used or in the duration of bleeding per period for either category of patients. The side effects reported (nausea, headache, diarrhoea, etc.) appeared to be evenly distributed between the ethamsylate and placebo treatment periods. Withdrawal from the trial was not associated with side effects.

The results of the third trial (Kasonde and Bonnar, 1975) do not support the conclusion that ethamsylate reduces menstrual blood loss. Twenty-five women complaining of excessive menstrual blood loss or using IUD were studied during six consecutive periods. By random allocation, 12 patients received treatment during the third and fourth cycle with ethamsylate and 13 with epsilon-aminocaproic acid (EACA). There was however a great difference in blood loss between the groups before treatment started (94.6 and 132.3 ml) and a great deal of variation within each group $(94.3 \pm 89.6$ and $59.8 \pm 46.7$, mean $\pm$ SD). Ethamsylate was taken as 500 mg tablets four times a day and EACA as a powder dissolved in water, 3 grams four times a day. Both treatments were administered from the onset of menstruation until bleeding ceased. Eleven women in each group completed the study. One of the two patients who dropped out from the EACA group did so after experiencing severe headaches during treatment. Blood loss was measured by photometrical readings of the iron pigment extracted from all sanitary towels used.

The average menstrual blood loss during the six consecutive cycles in the ethamsylate group did not vary significantly (ranging between 94.3 ml and 109.5 ml/cycle). In contrast, treatment with EACA was associated with a reduction of menstrual blood loss by almost 50% ($p<0.001$). It should be mentioned, however, that there was a great deal of variation in blood loss between groups both before treatment (e.g. 94.6 ± 73.6 ml – ethamsylate group; 132.3 ± 102.3 ml–EACA group) and during the trial (e.g. 94.3 ± 89.6 ml – ethamsylate group; 59.8 ± 46.7 ml – EACA group). Although all results were converted to logarithms before applying statistical analysis, it seems hazardous to draw any significant conclusions from these data. In comparison with the previously mentioned report (Campbell and Harrison, 1976), this study presents at least two important differences:
(1) women with and without IUD were considered together;
(2) treatment was limited to the days of menstruation. Whether these differences can account for the opposite results obtained is not known.

## Clinical efficacy in individuals without a bleeding disorder

A number of clinical trials have been performed to evaluate the haemostatic effect of ethamsylate on patients undergoing different types of surgical intervention.

Unfortunately, no study has fully conformed to the requirements for clinical trials recommended by the organizers of the Leuven meeting. Some of them, however, are worth mentioning.

*Tonsillectomy.* Five clinical trials were designed to evaluate the effect of ethamsylate on blood loss occurring during and/or after tonsillectomy. Three of them (de Reynier, 1965; Papatheodosslou, 1973; Verstraete *et al.*, 1977) were conducted in a controlled double-blind way, and bleeding was measured by an objective method (haemoglobin). Two of these 3 studies claimed a favourable effect of ethamsylate pretreatment in reducing intraoperative blood loss but the recent double-blind trial of Verstraete *et al.* (1977) did not. De Reynier (1965) reported that 12 patients on placebo had an average blood loss of 213 ml (range 94-445 ml), whereas in the 12 patients on ethamsylate the average blood loss was 155 ml (range 77-320 ml). Papatheodosslou (1973) found a mean blood loss of 27.5 ml in 100 patients receiving the placebo treatment, and of 4.8 ml in 100 patients given ethamsylate. Both values are much lower than the value of 165 ml indicated by the same author as the mean blood loss of untreated normal subjects undergoing tonsillectomy.

Neither de Reynier (1965) nor Papatheodosslou (1973) randomly allocated their patients to placebo or drug treatment. In addition, the inclusion and exclusion criteria used to select the patients were not mentioned in detail and there was no attempt to demonstrate that the control and the treated groups were equal at the start with respect to factors which were possibly relevant in determining the bleeding severity at operation. Finally, the results were not analyzed statistically.

The trial designed by Verstraete *et al.* (1977) to assess the efficacy of ethamsylate in adenotonsillectomy was a prospective, randomized, controlled double-blind study comprising 100 patients at the start. Nine patients were not included in the final analysis for various reasons. There was no significant difference between the overall blood loss (4.21 ± 1.70 ml/kg) of the 30 adenotonsillectomy patients pretreated 15 min before operation with 250 mg ethamsylate intravenously and that (4.55 ± 1.69 ml/kg) of the 25 control patients of the same group. The conclusion was the same for the 15 patients who underwent adenoidectomy only and who were pretreated with ethamsylate and the 21 control patients of the adenoidectomy group (2.45 ± 1.68 and 2.89 ± 1.39 ml/kg, respectively).

The clinical studies by Fumeaux (1961) and by Gobin (1966) were open trials with control groups. The planning and carrying out of both trials and the analysis of the results were so poor that they are of no significance.

*Prostatic Resection.* Three clinical trials are available on the effect of ethamsylate on blood loss during and/or after resection of the prostate. All three indicate a haemostatic effect of this drug. However the open trial reported by Hachen (1965) did not fulfil any of the minimum criteria required by the Leuven meeting and will therefore not be discussed here. In contrast, the studies performed by Symes *et al.* (1975) and by Mackenny (1976) are of some interest. Symes *et al.* (1975) measured in an objective way the blood loss during and after transurethral resection for benign enlargement of the prostate in 87 patients. Eleven of these patients were subsequently found to have carcinoma in the tissue removed at operation and were excluded from the first analysis of the results. Sadly, treatment was allocated to the first 46 patients on a single blind basis, in alternating blocks of 10, whereas only the last 41 patients were allocated to placebo or drug treatment in a double-blind manner and in random order. Even more regrettable is the fact that analysis of the data was not carried out separately for the two differently allocated groups of patients. The authors state that when the effects of treatment on the first 46 patients were compared with those for the last 41, no change in trend could be detected. However, the results of this preliminary analysis are not given in the report. It seems of little value to us that the retrospective examination of the combined placebo or drug treatment group showed good matching with respect to age, blood pressure, blood urea, euglobulin clot lysis time and platelet count. Loss of blood at operation in the ethamsylate group was 17 ml as compared to 72 ml in the controls ($p < 0.001$). Postoperative blood loss was also lower in the patients treated with the drug (38 ml) than in the controls (103 ml) ($p < 0.05$). The significance of these results did not change when the blood loss was expressed as ml/g of prostate resected. Nine patients required blood transfusions: 7 in the placebo group and 2 in the treated group. Postoperative bleeding sufficiently severe to require returning the patient to theatre occurred in 1 patient who had been given ethamsylate.

No clinical evidence of deep vein thrombosis was found in either group. However, 2 of the 16 patients given ethamsylate and studied with [125]I labelled fibrinogen scanning showed clear evidence of calf thrombosis. A far larger series of patients and the concomitant study of a control group by this technique is needed to assess the potential postoperative thromboembolic risk associated with ethamsylate treatment.

Mackenney (1976) studied a small series of 30 patients to compare the effect of ethamsylate and of EACA as haemostatic agents when used in transvesical prostatectomy.

Ethamsylate was given first intravenously (50 mg) on induction of anaesthesia, and at a dosage of 250 mg every six hours for 48 hours, then orally at a dosage of 250 mg every six hours for 72 hours. The same treatment schedule was used for EACA (4 g). Control patients did not receive any haemostatic treatment.

Allocation of patients to one of the three groups was randomized. Blood loss was measured by counting the red blood cells present in the

24-hourly collected drainage fluid, for five days postoperatively. Notwithstanding a rather satisfactory performance of this trial, only general trends of efficacy and a qualitative evaluation of the two drugs could be obtained. EACA greatly reduced postoperative blood loss but increased the incidence of intravesical clot retention. Ethamsylate was less effective but still reduced the blood loss considerably. It also lowered the incidence of clot retention.

*Miscellaneous.* A single-blind trial claiming a favourable haemostatic effect of ethamsylate in proctological surgery (Arnous and Mot, 1966) cannot be given any weight due to its poor experimental design and to the subjective way of assessing the intensity of bleeding. The same serious limitations apply to a study conducted by Hypher and Carpenter (1968) on the effect of ethamsylate in cataract surgery and to a recent report by Cesany (1975) on the effect of the drug in plastic and reconstructive surgery.

Finally, a within-patient randomized comparison of the effects of ethamsylate and placebo in reducing haemorrhage following dental extraction (Robertson *et al.*, 1977) points to a marked haemostatic effect of the drug. This trial appears to have been well planned and conducted and the results carefully analysed. The criteria used to evaluate the effect, however, were not strictly objective.

## Side effects

No serious side effects attributable to the drug have been reported so far in patients treated with ethamsylate. Occasional nausea, headache or skin rash have been reported which disappeared when the dose was reduced.

## Recommended doses

250 or 500 mg tablets: adult dosage 500 mg, 3 or 4 times a day; paediatric dosage, 250 mg, 3 or 4 times a day. 250 mg ampoules (injectable i.m. or i.v.). For surgery or emergency use, a ready loaded disposable cartrix syringe is available containing 1 g ethamsylate in 2 ml. The dosage recommendation is 750 mg (1.5 ml) i.v. (or *per cannula*), followed if necessary by a further 0.5 ml during or at the end of operation.

## Conclusions

The mechanism of action of ethamsylate is still uncertain but it appears to be associated with its capacity to shorten the bleeding time. It has been suggested that both platelets and the vessel wall are modified by this drug in such a way that reduction of bleeding ensues.

From a clinical point of view, ethamsylate seems to be an effective haemostatic drug in primary menorrhagia and possibly in patients undergoing prostatectomy, dental extraction or adenotonsillectomy. Particularly for the latter three conditions, further studies are required before firm conclusions can be reached. Evidence for the efficacy of ethamsylate in reducing bleeding associated with an IUD is contradictory. Claims for a beneficial effect of ethamsylate in reducing bleeding in uraemic patients undergoing peritoneal dialysis or in patients undergoing various types of surgical intervention are not substantiated by any well conducted clinical trials. No serious side effects seem to be attributable to treatment with ethamsylate. However, the potential thromboembolic risk associated with such a treatment has not been carefully assessed.

More studies on the kinetics, metabolism and bioavailability of the drug (when given orally or parenterally) in man are also desirable. This information may be of crucial importance in establishing rational treatment schedules. The interaction of ethamsylate with the other drugs most commonly used in patients with actual or potential bleeding disorders should also be investigated.

REFERENCES

ARNOUS J. and MOT J.C. (1966) Essais d'un nouvel hémostatique de synthèse la Dicynone, en chirurgie proctologique. *Agressologie* 7, 265.
BIZZI B., DONATI M.B. and DE GAETANO G. (1970) Ricerche sull' effetto emostatico della ciclonamina. *Gazz. int. Med. Chir.* 75, 501.
CAGIANELLI M.A., VILLANI C. and MIRENDA P. (1968) Su alcuni aspetti della sindrome emorragica del cirrotico. (Modificazioni dell'adesività piastrinica da Ciclononamina). *Boll. Soc. med. chir. Pisa* 36, 271.
CAJOZZO A., CITARRELLA P. and MALLEO C. (1973) Ulteriori osservazioni sulla attività capillaro-trofica dell'etanisilato in soggetti con turbe dell'emostasi di varia natura. *Gazz. med. ital.* 132, 200.
CAMPBELL S. and HARRISON R. (1976) A double-blind trial of ethamsylate (Dicynene) in the treatment of excessive menstrual bleeding in patients with and without intrauterine contraceptive devices. *Lancet* ii, 283.
CANAL P. (1964) Ensayo comparativo de la accion de la ciclonamina y un placebo. *Anales del Hospital de la Santa Cruz y San Pablo* 24, 253.
CESANY P. (1975) Etude clinique sur l'efficacité de la cyclonamine (Dicynone®) en chirurgie plastique et reconstructive. *Boll. Med. Svizz. ital.* 40, 3547.

COCCONI G. (1968) Dihydroxybenzenesulfonate de diethylammonium ou cyclonamine (Dicynone). In: *Compte-Rendu de la Société Italienne de Médecine Interne, Rome 13-16 Oct.*, pp. 526-528.

DAUBRESSE J.-C. (1971) Etamsylate et fragilité capillaire chez le diabétique. *Rev. méd. Liège* 26, 511.

DEACOCK A.R. de C. and BIRLEY D.M. (1969) The anti-haemorrhagic activity of ethamsylate (Dicynene). *Brit. J. Anaesth.* 41, 18.

de REYNIER J.-P. (1965) L'influence de la prémédication au Dicynone® sur le volume de la perte de sang durant l'amygdalectomie. *Praxis* 52, 1594.

FUMEAUX J. (1961) Etude clinique de l'activité d'un antihémorragique dérivé de la cyclohexadiénolone. *Rev. thérap.* 2, 1.

GOBIN (1966) Complications hémorragiques post-opératoires après amygdalo-adenoidectomie chez le nourrisson ou chez l'enfant. *Cahiers d'O.R.L.* 1, 103.

GUIDICELLI C. (1969) Thèse pharm., Montpellier.

HACHEN H.J. (1965) Contribution à la recherche expérimentale et clinique de l'action hémostatique du Dicynone®. *De Med. Tuenda* 3, 65.

HUGUET G., THOMAS J. and RAYNAUD G. (1969) Action d'un hémostatique, la cyclonamine, sur la perméabilité et la résistance capillaires. Etude complémentaire. *Thérapie* 24, 429.

HYPHER T. and CARPENTER R. (1968) Cyclonamine in cataract surgery: A clinical trial. *Brit. J. Ophthal.* 52, 375.

JACOBS A. and BUTLER E.B. (1965) Menstrual blood-loss in iron-deficiency anaemia. *Lancet* ii, 407.

JAFFE G. and WICKHAM A. (1973) A double-blind pilot study of Dicynene in the control of menorrhagia. *J. int. med. Res.* 1, 127.

KASONDE J.M. and BONNAR J. (1975) Effect of ethamsylate and aminocaproic acid on menstrual blood loss in women using intrauterine devices. *Brit. med. J.* iv, 21.

LOUIS J. and PAULUS J.M. (1967) Essai d'un nouvel hémostatique: la Dicynone. *Rev. méd. Liège* 22, 649.

MACKENNEY P.P. (1976) Post-prostatectomy bleeding and the use of haemostatic drugs. *J. roy. coll. Surg. Edinb.* In press.

MEDD R.H., CLIFFORD R., STREET A.E. and PRENTICE D.E. (1976) The effect of ethamsylate on the generalized Schwartzman reaction in rabbits. *Haematologica*. In press.

MARIGNAN R., CHANAL J.L., and GUIDICELLI C. (1967) Study of the decay of blood concentration with $C^{14}$ labelled Dicynene. *Soc. Pharmacol. Montpellier*, 27, 29.

MIGNE J., DEBADIER P. and RABY C. (1967) Methode d'étude de l'adhésivité plaquettaire in vitro par thrombélastographie, ses modifications sous l'influence d'agents thérapeutiques. In: *Proc. 10th Congr. Europ. Soc. Haemat., Strasbourg, 1965*. Part 2, pp. 1134-1141, Karger, Basel.

ORLANS F.B. (1973) Population Report, Series B., no. 1, Washington University Medical Centre.

PAPATHEODOSSLOU N. (1973) Essai de la Dicynone en double aveugle dans des cas d'amygdalectomies. *Méd. et Hyg. (Genève)* 31, 1818.

PRATO V. and FIORINA L. (1968) Richerche cliniche e rilievi sperimentali sull'attività antiemorragica del cicloesadienolone (Dicynone). *Minerva med.* 59, 1653.

RABY C. and COUPIER J. (1965) Nouvel hémostatique et antihémorragique de synthèse. In: *C.R. Xe Congr. Soc. Int. Transfusion Sanguine, Stockholm, 1964*. Vol. 5, pp. 1-7, Karger, Basel.

ROBERTSON C.J., ARBUCKLE J.M., BLAIR J., HENDERSON G.M., SYKES P. and OLIVANT J.M. (1977) Multi-centre trial of Dicynene in dental surgery. Submitted for publication.

Symes J.M., Offen D.N., Lyttle J.A., Blandy J.P. and Chaput De Saintonge D.M. (1975) The effect of Dicynene on blood loss during and after transurethral resection of the prostate. *Brit. J. Urol.* 47, 203.

Verstraete M., Tyberghein J., De Greef Y., Daems L. and Van Hoof A. (1977) Double-blind trials with ethamsylate, Batroxobin or tranexamic acid on blood loss after adenotonsillectomy. *Acta clin. belg.* 32., 136.

# Comments by the manufacturer of Dicynene®

by J.V. Reed, Delandale Laboratories Limited, Canterbury, Kent

With regard to brand names, Dicynene® is also known as Dicynone®. The name cyclonamine is I believe an alternative generic name and has not been used as a brand name as far as I know. Earlier papers also refer to 141E, 141MD, the two laboratory numbers which it has had at various stages. Although some earlier workers considered that ethamsylate was related to Congo Red, it seems to me that there is very little resemblance between the chemistry of ethamsylate and that of Congo Red, beyond the fact that benzene rings are involved. I notice also that Naphthionin® is stated to be related to Congo Red and that in the reference list to Naphthionin®, appear Estève and Regne, two authors who had a good deal to do with the early development of ethamsylate. My suspicion is that the finding of some haemostatic action in Congo Red may well have been the stimulus to research molecules for haemostatic action, but I think it is carrying it a bit far to suggest that Dicynene® is in any way derived from Congo Red.

The multicentre dental study of Robertson *et al.* was planned as a double-blind trial but, whilst the ampoules were supposed to be unidentifiable, there was in fact a clear difference between the ethamsylate and saline placebo ampoules; this paper is submitted for publication.

Concerning the i.v. administration of ethamsylate, it should be born in mind that when high molecular weight plasma volume expanders (e.g. dextrans) are being used, ethamsylate should be administered before these, not after. This is because dextran apparently absorbs the ethamsylate molecule and renders it ineffective if the substances are given in the wrong order.

# Report on aminaphtone[1]

## Chemistry

Aminaphtone is 2-hydroxy 3-methyl-1,4 naphthohydroquinone-2- (p-aminobenzoate). Molecular weight: 309.33.

## Mode of action

The mode of action is not known. It is believed to be a 'vasoactive' drug and to normalize abnormal capillary permeability. It does not induce platelet aggregation and does not alter blood coagulation (Fusco and Ross, 1975; De Pina-Cabral, 1973).

## Animal and human pharmacology

In rabbits, aminaphtone is excreted in the urine, mainly in the oxidized form. When the drug was given orally, 70-80% of the administered dose (100 mg/kg) was recovered in the urine between 58 and 144 hours (Pepeu, 1975).

No data are available about its absorption and metabolism in man.

The toxicology of aminaphtone has been studied by Pepeu (1975) in mice, rats, rabbits and dogs. From these experiments it appears that the drug has a very low acute and long-term toxicity. No deaths or toxic symptoms were observed up to doses of 3.0 g/kg aminaphtone in rabbits, mice and rats. In dogs, a dose of 1.5 g/kg produced no toxic symptoms. Oral administration of aminaphtone to female rats up to a dose of 60 mg/kg had no effect on reproduction. No malformations were observed in the new-borns. At a dose of 500 mg/kg the number of pregnancies was strongly reduced, indicating an effect on the early phase

1. Capillarema®.

of reproduction. Spermatogenesis was not altered in male rats treated for 15 days with 60 mg/kg aminaphtone. Aminaphtone did not induce neoplasms in mice (Michelazzi, 1973).

## Efficacy

*Animal experiments.* The effect of aminaphtone upon bleeding time in rabbits and mice was studied by Pepeu (1975). His results indicate that in rabbits oral administration of aminaphtone significantly shortens the bleeding time. The minimal effective dose is 0.1 mg/kg. There is a direct dose-effect relationship from 0.1-0.3 mg/kg. Doses higher than 0.3 mg/kg do not shorten the bleeding time further, but the effect is prolonged. Following oral administration of 0.2 mg/kg the effect on the bleeding time lasts from 30 min to 4 h. Aminaphtone also significantly reduces the bleeding time in mice. A moderate tachyphylaxis but no inversion of the effect was observed. The prolongation of bleeding time after administration of heparin is prevented by pretreatment with aminaphtone. In rabbits, aminaphtone reduces the immunological haemorrhagic weal caused by injection of antiplatelet serum and prevents the development of 5-hydroxytryptamine.

From these experiments it can be concluded that aminaphtone is able to shorten the bleeding time in rabbits and mice.

*Effect of aminaphtone upon bleeding time in humans.* A systematic study on the effect of aminaphtone on bleeding time and bleeding intensity was performed by Tammaro *et al*. (1973). The authors administered 150 mg aminaphtone orally per day for six days to 40 patients with various haemorrhagic diseases. 12 patients received a placebo. Bleeding time (Duke), bleeding intensity (de Nicola and Candura, 1961) and capillary fragility were determined before and during treatment. The authors claim that the drug shortened the bleeding time significantly and reduced the bleeding intensity, while the placebo was without effect.

This study does not fulfil the criteria of an adequate clinical trial for several reasons:
(1) The selection of the patients for the study was not restrictive enough. The patients included in the study had a wide variety of diseases; some had clotting defects (haemophilia) or platelet disorders (throm-

bocytopenia), others had haematological diseases, hepatic disorders or acute gastrointestinal bleeding without haemostatic defect. Many of these patients had acute conditions (acute hepatitis, acute bleeding) where the situation can change very rapidly. Therefore, a change in bleeding time may occur spontaneously and is not necessarily due to the action of the drug. It was not stated whether these patients received any other treatment (which might be expected).

(2) The patients were not randomly allocated to the treatment or the placebo group. The distribution of the various diseases between the treatment and placebo groups is unequal.

(3) It was not stated whether the study was performed double-blind.

(4) The authors did not state how long after the beginning of the treatment with aminaphtone the second test was performed (after six days ?).

In view of these facts the results of this study should be interpreted with great caution. On the other hand, the effects described in the treatment group are so striking and uniform, that it appears likely that the drug really has the effect claimed by the authors. Confirmation by a new trial, meeting all the requirements of a clinical trial is, however, necessary.

*Clinical efficacy. Prophylactic treatment.* Aliboni *et al*. (1972) studied the antihaemorrhagic effect of aminaphtone in patients undergoing tooth extraction. 152 patients received 2 mg/kg aminaphtone on the evening of the day preceeding the intervention and the same dose on the morning of the day of tooth extraction. This group was compared to 222 untreated patients. The presence or absence of bleeding was judged 2 h, 8 h and 24 h after the intervention, by the surgeon, who did not know to which group the patient belonged. The patients had no haemostatic abnormalities.

Compared to the untreated group, patients pretreated with aminaphtone showed significantly fewer haemorrhagic complications ($\chi^2$ test).

The experimental model used by the authors is quite interesting and is certainly suitable for testing the efficacy of a haemostatic agent. Further, the study has the advantage that the judgement of bleeding was done by a doctor who had no knowledge of the patient pretreatment. Unfortunately, in many other details the design of the study was not in accordance with the requirements of a clinical trial:

(1) The treatment group was compared only with an untreated group (no placebo group).
(2) There was no random allocation of the patients to the two groups and it is obvious from the figures that the groups are not comparable e.g. with regard to the type of anaesthesia and probably with regard to age, sex, or number of extracted teeth.
(3) There was no objective method for measuring blood loss following tooth extraction. The results are based only on clinical impression. It must be admitted, however, that in this special case it would be very difficult to measure the blood loss accurately using an objective method.

The same authors have performed a second small study including 21 patients who had a history of bleeding or had abnormal results of coagulation tests. All these patients were treated prophylactically with aminaphtone and the authors stated that no bleeding occured in these patients. The same objections as mentioned above must be made against this second study.

Jürgens (1969, 1970) treated prophylactically with aminaphtone a large number of patients with various bleeding disorders such as haemophilia, von Willebrand-Jürgens-syndrome, thrombopathia and thrombocytopenia. He stated that during treatment, haemorrhagic symptoms such as haematomas or nose bleeds were absent or less frequent compared to a period prior to treatment. These favourable results were based, however, only on clinical impressions. Except in a small group of haemophiliacs, no attempt was made to study the prophylactic effect of aminaphtone systematically.

Jürgens (1969) compared the bleeding frequency in a group of haemophiliacs before and during administration of aminaphtone. He claimed that the number of joint haemorrhages, of bleeding into the soft tissues and from the nasopharyngeal space were greatly reduced during treatment with 150 mg aminaphtone daily. Unfortunately no details about the patients who had been included in the study, or how the trial was conducted were given. It seems that there was no control group (each patient served as his own control). An objective measure for the degree of bleeding tendency before and during treatment is lacking (e.g. the number of hospital admissions, the units of factor VIII required for treatment of spontaneous haemorrhages, or the number of days lost from school or work). No statistical analysis was performed.

The data of Jürgens does not allow any conclusion as to the clinical efficacy of aminaphtone as a haemostatic agent.

## Side effects

None of the published papers mention side effects of aminaphtone. However it seems that a systematical attempt to look for certain possible side effects (e.g. stomach troubles, haedache) was not made in some trials. There is satisfactory evidence regarding the influence of treatment on hepatic, renal or bone marrow function.

## Recommended dose

For prophylatic treatment in man a dose of 2.5 mg/kg/24 h is recommended. (= 1 capsule of 25 mg per 10 kg body weight) (Jürgens, 1974).

## Conclusions

From pharmacological studies it seems to be proved that aminaphtone shortens the bleeding time in rabbits and mice.
It is possible that the drug might shorten the bleeding time and reduce the bleeding intensity in patients with various haemorrhagic diseases, but this has not yet been definitely proved by means of an adequate trial.
Several authors had the clinical impression that prophylactic treatment with aminaphtone reduces the frequency of spontaneous bleeding in patients with abnormal haemostasis. It is also claimed that postoperative bleeding is less frequent or less servere in aminaphtone-treated patients with normal or abnormal haemostasis. This clinical impression has still to be confirmed by controlled randomized trials.

REFERENCES

ALIBONI E., AMATO G. and MARINI A. (1972) Valutazione clinica dell'attivita' di un cappilaro-protettore. *Clin. odonto-protes.* 28, 59.
FUSCO F.A. and ROSSI E. (1975) L'impiego dell'aminaftone nelle sindromi emorragiche considerazione in base allo studio di determinati parimetri emocoagulativi. *Quad. Coagul.* 1, 5.

JURGENS J. (1970) Clinical practice in the bleeding prophylaxis of thrombocytogenic haemorrhagic diatheses using the haemostatic preparation 'aminaphton'. *Quad. Coagul.* 14, 1.

JURGENS J. (1969) Prophylaxe hämophiler Blutungen. In: *'Hämophilie', 11 Hamburger Symposion uber Blutgerinnung.* (Thies H. A. and Landbeck G., eds.), pp. 227-240.

MICHELAZZI L. (1973) Relazione biologica sopra la eventuale attivita cancerogena dell' 'Aminaftone'. *Quad. Coagul.* 15, 26.

DE NICOLA and CANDURA M.D. (1961) Etude de l'intensité du saignement dans la determination du temps de saignement. *Hémostase* 1, 113.

PEPEU G. (1975) Toxicological and pharmacological investigations on aminaphtone (2-hydrosy-3-methyl-1,4-naphthohydroquinone-2-aminobenzoate). *Quad. Coagul.* 1, 19.

DE PINA-CABRAL J.M. (1973) Result of Capillarema administration to dogs previously treated with a coumarin derivative. *Quad. Coagul.* 15, 32.

TAMMARO A.E., GIAROLA P.A. and BARTOLI G. (1973) Ricerche sull'azione antihemorragica dell'Aminaphtone. *Quad. Coagul.* 15, 38.

# Comments by the manufacturer of Capillarema®

**by U. Baldacci, Laboratori Baldacci, Pisa**

Aminaphtone is the generic name of 2-hydroxymethyl-1,4-naphthohydroquinone-2- (p-aminobenzoate), $C_{18} H_{15} O_4 N$.
The molecular weight is 309.33 and the structural formula is:

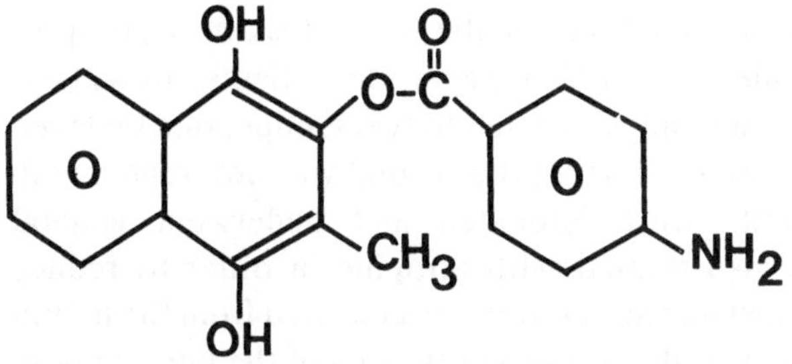

Aminaphtone is insoluble in water, soluble in acetone, ethanol and propylene glycol, and very sparingly soluble in ether, chloroform and benzene.

The efficacy of aminaphtone has recently been confirmed by animal and clinical experiments.

## Animal experiments

Table 1 shows that aminaphtone antagonizes the increase in bleeding time induced by heparin in rabbits.

The bleeding time was determined by the method of Roskam and Pauwen (1937).

The effect of aminaphtone (0.2 mg/kg p.o.) on the bleeding time (s) was determined on both ears of rabbits previously treated with heparin (4 mg per kg body weight administered intravenously).

*Table 1.* Effect of aminaphtone on the bleeding time of rabbits treated with heparin.

| | Number of experiments | Time after i.v. administration of heparin (min) | | | p between the bleeding time at 0 min and 30 min |
|---|---|---|---|---|---|
| | | 0 | 10 | 30 | |
| Carboxymethyl cellulose 1% | 6 | 111 ± 3.2 | 141 ± 11.1 | 143 ± 3.7 | p<0.01 |
| Aminaphtone | 6 | 114 ± 10.2 | 115 ± 10.0 | 96 ± 2 | p<0.01 |

## Clinical experiments

Amato *et al.* (in press) investigated quantitatively and with a double-blind procedure the effect of aminaphtone on the blood loss in a group of patients of both sexes undergoing oral surgery. The patients, all without bleeding disorders, were randomly allocated to two groups; one received aminaphtone *per os* 2 mg/kg for 4 days; the second was not treated with aminaphtone. All patients were intubated and underwent general anaesthesia; they were also treated with atropine in order to reduce salivation. All the blood lost during surgery was collected from the mouth by suction and its volume was determined at the end of the intervention. The results are reported in Table 2.

*Table 2.* Volume of blood lost during oral surgery.

| Treatment | Number of patients | Blood volume (ml) | |
|---|---|---|---|
| none | 15 | 36.7 ± 4.2 | |
| | | | p<0.05 |
| Aminaphtone 2 mg/kg p.o. ×4 days | 15 | 24.7 ± 3.6 | |

Aminaphtone brought a statistically significant decrease of the blood loss.

## Side Effects

Haematological investigations and liver function tests were carried out on patients treated with aminaphtone and the reports submitted to the Italian Ministry of Health in order to obtain the licence for marketing the compound. No toxic effects were observed.

Jürgens (1969) reported no side effects in patients with haemorrhagic disorders treated with aminaphtone for periods of time of a year or more.

Tammaro et al. (1970) mentioned that in 40 patients treated with aminaphtone for 6 days no side effects were observed.

Aminaphtone has been on the market in Italy since 1972 and no side effects have been reported.

REFERENCES

AMATO G., POLLINI C., MARINI A. and ALIBONI E. (1977) Studio sull'azione antiemorragica dell'aminaftone. Minerva Stomatol. In press.
JURGENS J. (1969) Prophylaxe hämophiler Blutungen. In: 'Hämophilie', 11 Hamburger Symposium uber Blutgerinnung. (Thies H. A. and Landbeck G., eds.), pp. 227-240.
ROSKAM J. and PAUWEN L. (1937) Une technique et une méthode pour l'étude de l'hémostase spontanée et des médications hémostatiques. Arch. int. Pharmacodyn. 59, 450.
TAMMARO A., GIAROLA P.A. and BARTOLI G. (1973) Ricerche sull' azione antiemorragica dell' aminaftone. Quad. Coagul. 5, 38.

# Report on a preparation of pectin[1]: Sangostop®

Sangostop® was introduced as a haemostatic agent in 1935 by Brahn *et al.* (1935) and by Reisser and Nagel (1935). It was stated that it could reduce all kinds of bleeding and could be administered locally, by mouth, intramuscularly, subcutaneously or *per rectum.*

## Chemical composition

The active component consists of colloidal polygalacturonic acid esters from apple pectin. The solution for local and oral use contains 5% pectin (colloidal polygalacturonic acid esters 5%, calcium chloride 0.7%); the solution for injection, 3% pectin (colloidal polygalacturonic acid esters 3%, calcium chloride 0.5%, sodium chloride 0.7%). The pH of the solution is 3.6-3.8.

## Mode of action

In 1924 Violle and de Saint-Rat in France were the first to report on the haemostatic effect of pectin. They used a 1 or 2% solution of pectin and found that as much as 50 ml per kg body weight, administered orally, could be given to rabbits without any injury. In a later paper Violle and de Saint-Rat (1925) contended that it was the pectin itself and not the products of disintegration that were effective. Feissly (1925) used a 1% pectin sol, to which he added calcium chloride and sodium chloride and then autoclaved the mixture for 20 minutes at 120°C. He found that when given intravenously to rabbits or man this sol accelerated coagulation, whereas in dogs it had the opposite effect. Added *in vitro* to human blood, pectin was found to delay coagulation. Reisser and Nagel (1935)

1. Other similar preparations: Strypturon®, Arhémapectine®.

found that pectin (tetragalacturonic acid ester) had no effect on the coagulation of blood *in vitro*. In rabbits subcutaneous or intravenous infusion of pectin sols shortened the coagulation time, and this effect lasted for several hours. These authors pointed out that the neutral salts of polygalacturonic acid had no effect. They contended that the effect of these small amounts of acids was due to the irritation of the vessel endothelium at the site of passage of the acid into the blood. They felt that coagulative substances, probably thrombokinase, formed as a result of this irritation. Other workers (Brahn *et al.,* 1935; Baumann, 1937; Marx, 1939) also reported that Sangostop® or pectins shortened the coagulation time within 1 hour after parenteral infusion both in rabbits and in man. Marx (1939) found that serum from rabbits which had been given injections of pectin clotted a fibrinogen solution more rapidly than serum from untreated animals. Beller (1951) reported that Sangostop® had no effect on the prothrombin time in rabbits or in man, but that it did shorten the coagulation time for 30-50 minutes. Fleischhacker (1937) administered 'Liquoid' to rabbits to delay coagulation. After injection of pectin the coagulation times again became normal. Dietrich and Oettel (1937) found that pectin not only shortened the coagulation time, but also increased the platelet count and shortened the bleeding time.

From all these earlier studies it is clear that the mode of action of pectin on the haemostatic mechanism *in vivo* was unclear. No effect of pectin on coagulation *in vitro* could be detected.

In 1960 Fearnley *et al.* showed that beer and wine lowered the blood fibrinolytic activity. Nilsson *et al.* (1961) also found that the consumption of wine or beer, but not of ethyl alcohol, lowered the fibrinolytic activity of the blood. *In vitro* experiments showed that wine and beer contained a principle that inhibited fibrinolytic activators. This principle was isolated from grape pulp, and analysis showed it to be a pectin-like substance. In this connection they investigated different types of pectins and also Sangostop®. The antiactivator activity of the pectins was assayed by incubation with a solution of pig heart activator or urokinase solution and determination of the degree of inhibition produced. The samples were assayed for residual activator activity on unheated fibrin plates (see Nilsson *et al.,* 1961). A 3% solution of Sangostop® had an antiactivator activity corresponding to about twice that of undiluted red wine. Compared with ε-aminocaproic acid (EACA) the inhibitory effect of

Sangostop® corresponded to a solution containing 20 mg EACA per ml. The effect of Sangostop® on fibrinolysis *in vivo* was not studied.

## Animal and human pharmacology

No systematic pharmacological or toxicological studies are available. The drug has been reported to be effective on intravenous and intramuscular administration when given in doses of 10-30 ml of a 5% solution in man. The effect of one dose has been reported to last from 1 to several hours, as judged from the shortening of the coagulation time (see Joseph, 1940). When given by mouth the drug has no effect on the coagulation time (Fleischhacker, 1937). Neither the concentration of pectin in the blood nor its disappearance rate has been determined.

No toxic effects of the drug have been reported in animals or in man. As pointed out above, Violle and de Saint-Rat stressed, as early as 1924, that pectins in doses of 1 g per kg body weight caused no injury in rabbits. Aragona (1936) showed that prolonged oral administration of pectins to rabbits caused no gross or microscopic lesions. Brahn *et al.* (1935) gave rabbits 100 ml of a 2.5% solution of pectins, but observed no signs of lesions.

Judging from the literature (see Joseph, 1940) Sangostop® has been administered to a large number of patients, and all authors stress that the drug is completely non-toxic. Gohrbandt (1936) gave it to more than 400 patients and stressed that no thrombotic complications were seen.

However, no toxicological studies filling modern requirements are available.

## Clinical studies

The earlier literature contains several reports on the clinical usefulness of Sangostop® as a haemostatic agent for all types of bleeding. Gohrbandt (1936) published a report on the use of Sangostop® in more than 400 cases in connection with surgery. He found that it was an excellent haemostatic and that the bleeding decreased in all cases except one. Kochs (1935) found the treatment useful in lung bleeding, ulcerative colitis and for bleeding in the oral and nasal cavities. Sack (1935) used the pectin preparation for treatment of patients with gastric, pulmonary, renal, bladder and intestinal haemorrhages. He also reported that the treatment was effective in 3 patients with haemophilia. Dietrich and Oettel (1937) found that the drug was effective in patients with thrombocytopenia. Berberich (1936) published data on the use of Sangostop® in bleedings from the nose, ear and throat. He said that the drug was very effective, but he did not give the number of cases treated. He also said that if the drug was given before tonsillectomy, it could prevent postoperative bleeding. These results were not confirmed by Jongkees (1939), who gave the drug orally. Berberich administered the drug intramuscularly. Fleischhacker (1937), Langer and Hondelink (1937), Van Luyk (1938) and Almay (1938) also recommended the prophylactic use of Sangostop® before tonsillectomy, tooth extraction and adenoidectomy, to prevent postoperative bleeding. Roemer (1937) and also Fonyo (1938) found the drug useful in gynaecological bleeding.

Baumann (1937) reported excellent results with Sangostop® in 110 patients with abnormal bleeding conditions, excluding true haemophilia. He particularly studied the dosage problems. His conclusion was to give 20 ml Sangostop® i.m. 24 hours before operation, then 10 ml i.m. 4 hours before operation and to follow this orally with 5 tablespoons of the 5% solution 2 hours before operation.

The benefits of pectin as a haemostatic agent have thus been observed in a wide variety of bleeding situations, but in most cases the effect was judged subjectively only. Controlled clinical trials with or without quantitation of blood loss are not available.

## Conclusions

The active principle in Sangostop® is pectin. The haemostatic effect of pectin was earlier not understood, but it is known that pectins inhibit *in vitro* fibrinolytic activators. The benefits of pectin as a haemostatic agent have been observed in a great variety of bleeding situations, above all, in bleeding from the mucosa and postoperative bleeding. The effect has been judged subjectively only and no controlled clinical trials are available. No toxic effects have been reported but no critical toxicological investigations have been performed. The pharmacodynamics and pharmacokinetics of Sangostop® have not been investigated.

The investigations on record do not meet any of the requirements necessary for recognition of Sangostop® as a haemostatic. In view of the fact that Sangostop® contains pectin and thus of the possibility that it might act as an inhibitor of fibrinolysis, further investigation might be of interest.

## REFERENCES

ALMAY K. (1938) Application of Sangostop® in cases of profuse bleeding after teeth extraction. *Orv. Hetil.* 82, 529.

ARAGONA G. (1936) The time of coagulation of blood after the administration of the pectin to rabbits. *Boll. Soc. ital. Biol. sper.* 11, 434.

BAUMANN E. (1937) Experimentelle und klinische Untersuchungen über blutstillende Wirkung van Sangostop und Vitamin C. *Bruns' Beitr. klin. Chir.* 166, 298.

BELLER F.K. (1951) Über die Therapie bei Blutungen. *Therapiewoche* 10, 1.

BERBERICH J. (1936) Hemostasis by means of Sangostop in throat-nose-ear medical science. *Mschr. Ohrenheilk.* 70, 966.

BRAHN B., KLARENBEEK A. and LANGNER T. (1935) Onderzoek over een nieuw bloedstollingsmiddel. *Ned. T. Geneesk.* 37, 4362.

DIETRICH S. and OETTEL H. (1937) Treatment of blood diseases with pectin. *Dtsch. med. Wschr.* 65, 1690.

FEARNLEY G.R., FERGUSON J., CHAKRABARTI R. and VINCENT C.T. (1960) Effect of beer on blood fibrinolytic activity. *Lancet* i, 184.

FEISSLY R. (1925) Action of pectin on the coagulation of the blood. *C.R. Soc. Biol. (Paris)* 92, 317.

FLEISCHHACKER H. (1937) On the coagulating promotion of pectin. *Fortschritte der Therapie (Leipzig)* 13, 377.

FONYO J.L. (1938) Treatment of uterine atony and hemorrhage with new medicaments: vitamin C, vitamin P, pectin substances and manetol. *Gyógyaszat (Budapest)* 78, 284, 286, 302, 320.

GOHRBANDT E. (1936) The action of pectin as a blood coagulant. *Dtsch. med. Wschr.* 62, 1625.

JONGKEES, L.B.W. (1939) Hemostatic drugs as prophylactics in tonsillectomy and adenectomy. *Ned. T. Geneesk.* 83, 4640.

JOSEPH G.H. (1940) Medical literature on pectin and pectin pastes. *Bull. nat. Formulary Comm.* 9, 2.

KOCHS H. (1935) A pectin derivative as a blood coagulant and contribution for the control of colitis ulcerosa. *Münch. med. Wschr.* 82, 1284.

LANGNER T. and HONDELINK H. (1937) Objective and subjective data obtained in the clinical application of Sangostop in ear, nose and throat practice. *Ned. T. Geneesk.* 81, 188.

MARX R. (1939) *Beitrag zur experimentellen Untersuchung des Mechanismus der Wirkung von Pektin auf Blutgerinnung und Blutstillung und zum Studium des Verhaltens von Pektin im Stoffwechsel.* Thesis, University of Munich.

NILSSON I.M., BJORKMAN S.E., V. STUDNITE W. and HALLEN A. (1961) Antifibrinolytic activity of certain pectins. *Thrombos. Diathes. haemorrh. (Stuttg.)* 6, 177.

REISSER O. and NAGEL A. (1935) Über die gerinnungsfördernde Wirkung saurer Substanzen, insbesondere des Pektins. *Naunyn-Schmiedeberg's Arch. Pharmak. exp. Pathol.* 179, 748.

ROEMER H. (1937) Action and field of application of blood coagulation agents (Clauden, Manetol, Hamostatikum-Nordmark, and Sangostop). *Z. Geburtsh. Gynak.* 115, 230.

SACK G. (1935) The hemostyptic effect of pectins. Particularly in hemophilia. *Klin. Wschr.* 14, 1536.

VAN LUYK J.H.A. (1938) Sangostop in therapy of hemorrhage after teeth extraction. *Geneesk. Gids* 16, 1416.

VIOLLE H. and DE SAINT-RAT L. (1924) Pectin and its hemostatic effects. *C.R. Acad. Med.* 92, 1097.

VIOLLE H. and DE SAINT-RAT L. (1925) The hemostatic properties of pectin. *C.R. Acad. Sci. (Paris)* 180, 603.

# Report on naftazone[1]

## Chemistry

Naftazone is 1,2-naphthoquinone 2-semicarbazone.

$$\text{(structure)} = N - NH - C \underset{NH_2}{\overset{O}{\Big<}}$$

This compound, which was introduced by Derouaux (1961) is prepared by diazotization of sulphanilic acid with beta-naphthol; it is similar to adrenochrome which is also prepared in the stable monosemicarbazide form.

## Haemostatic action

The haemostatic action of naftazone appears very similar to that of adrenochrome.
(1) In a dose of 1 µg per kg, it reduces the bleeding time in the rabbit ear (technique of Roskam, 1933) by 30%.
(2) It apparently increases capillary resistance.
(3) It has no action on the levels of coagulation factors, and does not affect coagulation tests.

## Dosage

Presented as 1 mg tablets and ampoules containing 100 µg per 2 ml.

1. Haemostop®, Karbinone®.

## Toxicity

Toxicity in experimental animals is very low, and the $LD_{50}$ dose in mice of 27 g per kg, is identical to that produced by the solvent (La Barre and Gillo).

## Studies in experimental animals

Initial animal studies were carried out by Dermaut and Gilson (1963), who assessed the effect of naftazone in rabbits and dogs. In rabbits, prior injection of naftazone 1 µg/kg reduced the blood lost in an ear bleeding time technique from 112.4 g% to a mean of 40.4 g%, a reduction of 72 g%. There was also a significant drop from 34.8 g% to 26.8 g% loss following naftazone 2 µg/kg given intravenously to dogs in whom a mesenteric vessel had been severed. In man, naftazone significantly increased capillary resistance, as determined by the ventouse technique.

Naftazone also has a protective effect in rabbits (Laborit and Baron, 1971) and dogs (Dermaut and Gilson, 1963) subjected to experimental haemorrhagic shock. There was improved arterial blood pressure and an increased rate of survival in animals pretreated with naftazone. Laborit and Baron (1971) have suggested that the quinone molecule may play a protective role at intracellular level, as well as having a strengthening effect on capillary resistance.

## Controlled clinical studies

Charles and Coolsaet (1972) carried out a double-blind controlled clinical trial with naftazone or placebo in patients undergoing prostatectomy. Naftazone was started orally the evening prior to surgery, and continued by i.m. and i.v. routes during the period prior to, and during, surgery. Postoperatively, urinary blood loss was measured and blood transfusion requirements noted. Blood loss of 604 ml (mean) in the control group was significantly reduced to 314 ml in the treated group. Similarly, a mean of 600 ml blood was transfused in the control group against 342 ml in the treatment group. The authors considered 1.2-naphthoquinone to play an important role in the reduction of surgical blood loss.

Lambert and Abravanel (1970) used naftazone during tooth extraction.

In an initial study, 60 patients were divided into two groups of 30 (allocation method not stated). The treated patients all stopped bleeding within ten minutes (apart from one who bled for one hour). In the control patients, ten bled for periods of greater than ten minutes.

In the second study, ten patients who needed several extractions were treated first without and later with naftazone. In eight of the ten cases there was a shorter bleeding duration with naftazone. The authors were impressed by the haemostatic effect of naftazone.

Deuil (1972) used naftazone to determine whether the progress of diabetic retinopathy could be retarded. Fifty diabetic patients were divided into two groups (method of allocation not stated). The treatment group received 6 mg naftazone daily (two tablets three times daily) for fifteen months. At the final ophthalmic examination the following results were obtained:

|               | Total | Improved | Stationary | Worse |
|---------------|-------|----------|------------|-------|
| Treated group | 50    | 24       | 21         | 5     |
| Control group | 50    | 3        | 19         | 28    |

These are impressive results, and should be followed up by controlled trials, particularly as ophthalmic assessment is not an objective endpoint.

## Conclusions

There is not a great deal of controlled clinical data available on naftazone. Its mode of action appears to be similar to that of adrenochrome, but it may have important additional actions at the cellular level. Further controlled trials in the field of prostatic surgery, dental extraction and diabetic retinopathy would appear desirable before any definite recommendation for this drug can be made.

REFERENCES

CHARLES O. and COOLSAET B. (1972) Prevention des hémorragies en chirurgie prostatique. *Ann. Urol.* 6, 209.

DERMAUT G. and GILSON M. (1963) Etude expérimental des propriétés hémostatiques et de l'activité vasculaire de la monosemicarbazone de la beta-naphtoquinone. *Arch. int. Pharmacodyn.* 146, 517.

DEROUAUX G. (1961) Etude expérimentale des propriétés hémostatiques de la monosemicarbazone de la beta-naphtoquinone. *C.R. Soc. Biol. (Paris)* 155, 950.

DEUIL R. (1972) Histoire naturelle de la rétinopathie diabétique. Role de l'equilibre du diabète. *Gaz. méd. Fr.* 79, 1917.

LABORIT H. and BARON C. (1971) Effets de la monosemicarbazone de la beta-naphtoquinone dans le choc hémorragique expérimentale. *Agressologie* 12, 25.

LAMBERT A. and ABRAVANEL V. (1970) Traitement préventif des hémorragies en stomatologie. La monosemicarbazone de la bèta-naphtoquinone. *Acta stomat. belg.* 67, 365.

ROSKAM J. (1933) *C.R. Soc. Biol. (Paris)* 122, 1245.

# Comments by the manufacturer of Karbinone®

**by G. Derouaux, spokesman for Seresci, Brussels**

(1) There are two publications which support the protective effect of naftazone in haemorrhagic shock. (Dermaut and Gilson, 1963; Laborit and Baron, 1971).

(2) Winand (1977) has demonstrated an increase in various lysosomal enzymes in the walls of varicose veins and in the plasma of patients with varicose veins, and has observed a significant decrease in these same enzymes after treatment with naftazone. The action of naftazone is not due to an inhibitory action on the lysosomal enzymes but rather to a protective effect on the lysosome membranes.

(3) Naftazone was first introduced at a time when clinical trials were not as well defined and standardized as they are these days, and further, standardized trials would now probably be welcome. However, it must be emphasized that naftazone is a 'vascular haemostatic drug' which means that it does not modify any of the coagulation parameters (Dermaut and Gilson, 1963; Derouaux and Thouverez, 1969). The fact that it does not act at the level of the coagulation factors excludes the possibility that it will initiate disseminated intravascular coagulation.

The work by Winand (1977) on the protective effect of naftazone on the lysosomal membranes (see also Laborit and Baron, 1971) will no doubt throw some light on the 'vascular' action of naftazone.

REFERENCES

DERMAUT G. and GILSON M. (1963) Etude expérimentale des propriétés hémostatiques et de l'activité vasculaire de la monosemicarbazone de la β-naphtoquinone (S.C.B.N.). *Arch. int. Pharmacodyn.* 146, 517.

DEROUAUX G. and THOUVEREZ J.P. (1969) A propos de l'importance du facteur vasculaire dans l'hémostase. *Coagulation*, 2, 193.

LABORIT H. and BARON C. (1971) Effets de la monosemicarbazone de la β-naphtoquinone dans le choc hémorragique expérimental. *Aggressologie*, 1, 25.

WINAND R. (1977) La mono-semicarbazone 2 de la β-naphtoquinone (D.C.I. naftazone) dans la maladie variqueuse. *Rev. méd. Liège.* In press.

# Report on adrenochrome monosemicarbazide[1] (carbazochrome) and carbazochrome salicylate[2]

## Chemistry

Adrenochrome is an oxidation product of adrenaline (epinephrine) as shown by Green and Richter (1937). Both compounds are unstable, but Braconier *et al*. (1943) found that when adrenochrome is combined with monosemicarbazone the resulting compound adrenochrome monosemicarbazide (carbazochrome) is stable. This substance is poorly soluble but becomes much more soluble in the form of a sodium salicylate complex and can be given by intramuscular injection or orally. The official name for this compound is carbazochrome salicylate.

The formula of adrenochrome monosemicarbazone is:

$$NH_2-\overset{\overset{O}{\|}}{C}-NH-N=\quad\text{(ring structure)}\quad\overset{H}{\underset{}{C}}-OH,\ -CH_2,\ N-CH_3,\ O=$$

which can be compared with the parent molecule adrenaline.

There is evidence that adrenochrome may act, in some respects, as a precursor of adrenaline, distributed throughout the tissues, which is slowly converted to adrenaline within the body (Bacq *et al*., 1949).

Despite its adrenaline-like action on small blood vessels, adrenochrome does not give rise to the general systemic effects of sympathomimetic drugs.

1. Adona AC-17®, Adrenoxyl®, Emex®.
2. Adrenosem®.

## Theoretical mode of action of adrenochrome monosemicarbazone

(1) Adrenaline-like action
(2) Increases capillary resistance and promotes retraction of severed capillaries
(3) Reduces capillary permeability
(4) Shortens bleeding time
(5) Vitamin P-like action
(6) Adrenal stimulating effect

## Pharmacology

Carbazochrome salicylate can be given intramuscularly or orally. Oral absorption is approximately one-third that of intramuscular injection. Carbazochrome is rapidly oxidised in the body and eliminated within a 12-hour period. The monosemicarbazone is excreted from 50-70% through the kidneys, and 20-30% by means of indole formation.

## Mode of action as a haemostatic agent

The haemostatic action of carbazochrome and derivatives is said to be exerted solely in the capillaries. Capillary resistance is increased in both the guinea pig and man as demonstrated by the ventouse technique (Prevost, et al., 1947). These authors found that, in man, the bleeding time was reduced from a 'normal' value of 200 seconds to between 110-130 seconds one hour after carbazochrome (Adrenoxyl®) injection. The duration of effect appeared to be dose related in that after injection of 1 or 2 mg carbazochrome the effect lasted up to 6 hours, but that 4 to 6 mg produced an effect which lasted for 24 hours.

Prevost et al. (1947) also noted that the bleeding time was shortened in patients with an initially prolonged bleeding time, ranging from 300-1,260 seconds, although the cause of prolonged bleeding time was not stated. The bleeding time in these patients was reduced by from 60% to 30%. Roskam and Derouaux (1944) demonstrated that carbazochrome, given intravenously, intramuscularly or subcutaneously, shortened significantly the bleeding time in human volunteers for a period of up to two hours after treatment. These observations were confirmed by Duesberg (1947).

Herve and Lecomte (1949) have shown that the degree of ecchymosis induced in the skin of mice following irradiation can be reduced by pretreatment with adrenochrome. This reduction has been attributed to the effect of adrenochrome in increasing capillary resistance and diminishing capillary permeability.

Capillary permeability following experimental injury by hyaluronidase and snake venoms was reduced by prior administration of adrenochrome (Zweifach and Chambers, 1950).

*Vitamin P.* The action of adrenochrome in increasing capillary resistance has been ascribed to a vitamin P-like component.

*ACTH-like effect.* Adrenochrome has apparently a mild, adrenal stimulating action, as judged by the Thorn test, and as tested in the rat.

## Toxicity

Adrenochrome appears to be a remarkably non-toxic product. It is not associated with generalized sympathetic stimulation and there appears to be no tachycardia, hypertension or anxiety following its administration. The $LD_{50}$ in experimental animals is 183 mg per kg body weight.

There appear to be no cumulative effects.

## Administration of carbazochrome salicylate

Intramuscular injection or oral, as syrup or tablet.

Dosage.

Oral: 15 ml syrup (7.5 mg) 1 hour prior to haemostatic challenge.

i.m. injection: 2 ml (10 mg) 20 minutes prior to haemostatic challenge.

These doses can be repeated at two-hourly intervals if there is continued bleeding.

## Experimental studies in animals

Hagerty *et al.* (1951) assessed the effect of Adrenoxyl® (carbazochrome) on blood loss from experimental surgical incisions in the liver in dogs. Incisions were made first without drug administration and then 60 minutes after Adrenoxyl® 10 mg given i.m. The amount of blood lost was reduced by over 70 per cent in four of five dogs, but was increased in the fifth dog.

An attempt was made in a small study to assess the effect of Adrenoxyl® on surgical blood loss, but no conclusions could be drawn.

Ruddell (1958) confirmed that Adrenoxyl® significantly shortened the bleeding time following incisions of rabbit ear vessels.

Klemm and Bolton (1967) evaluated a variety of haemostatic agents, including carbazochrome on lip bleeding time, incision oozing time and clotting time in dogs. Carbazochrome was given in a dosage of 0.44 mg/kg intravenously. There was slight but significant reduction in the bleeding and clotting times as detected in these tests, compared with saline placebo, but the authors felt that a substantial effect in reduction of bleeding did not occur.

White *et al.* (1966) demonstrated that carbazochrome neither activated Hageman factor nor shortened the clotting time in dogs.

## Double-blind controlled trials in which accurate quantitation of blood loss was not carried out

Forman and Naylor (1964) carried out a double-blind controlled clinical trial of carbazochrome versus placebo in dental extractions. Five hundred patients received tablets of which 395 results were analysed. Analysis was by questionnaire returned by patients, who assessed subjectively the extent of blood loss in the first 24 hours after extractions. Seventy-nine patients on the active drug reported bleeding continuing for longer than one hour compared with 105 patients on placebo ($p < 0.05$). However the control group had had a mean of 2.2 teeth extracted, compared with 1.9 teeth in the drug-treated group. The authors concluded that the drug had little active value, and its effects failed to confirm previous enthusiastic reports.

Calnan and Innes (1958) did a randomized double-blind trial in 76 patients having plastic surgery. Thirty-nine patients were treated with

Adrenoxyl® and 37 patients had placebo. There was no significant difference in the amount of bleeding, as assessed by the surgeon, between the two groups.

Dykes and Anderson (1961) gave, in a double-blind study, carbazo-chrome to 91 patients prior to plastic surgical operations and placebo injections to 91 controls. There was no significant difference in blood loss, as evaluated by the surgeons, between the two groups.

Marcus and Spaet (1958) studied 44 patients undergoing thoracic surgery. Twenty-three received Adrenosem® (carbazochrome salicylate) intramuscularly during the operation, and 21 received placebo injections. There was no significant difference between the two drugs as evaluated by overall assessment of operative and postoperative bleeding.

Swan et al. (1961), assessed the effect of Adrenoxyl® in reduction of hyphaemia after cataract surgery. Eighty patients were divided into two groups of 40 by random allocation within pairs of patients. One group was given Adrenoxyl® 10 mg orally 8 hourly for the duration of hospital stay and 40 were given nothing. There was no difference in the incidence of postoperative hyphaemia between the groups.

Horne and Scott (1970) carried out a double-blind cross-over study in 26 patients having excessive bleeding associated with an intrauterine device. There was no significant reduction in bleeding at menstruation. However, between periods a total of 145 days/cycle was reduced to 93 days/cycle on Adrenosem®. The number of pads used during placebo periods was 103/cycle and during Adrenosem® 54/cycle. Thus, intermenstrual bleeding is significantly reduced by Adrenosem® treatment.

## Controlled studies with quantitation of blood loss but not random allocation

Durante et al. (1962) assessed the effect of several haemostatic agents, including Adrenosem®, on blood loss following prostatectomy. Blood loss was followed by haemoglobin estimations on all post-operative drainage and irrigating fluid collected by indwelling catheters. The effect of Adrenosem® was only assessed in four patients, and these appeared to lose more blood (average postoperative blood loss 304 ml) than the 27 control patients (average loss 75 ml) following transurethral resection.

Conversely, in a double-blind study Burke et al. (1960) found that post-operative bleeding after transurethral prostatectomy was reduced from 256 ml in 48 control cases to 68 ml in 14 Adrenosem® treated patients.

Thajeb *et al*. (1959) carried out a comparison of 1) Koagamin®, 2) carbazochrome (Adrenosem®) and 3) intravenous oestrogens (Premarin®) to reduce postoperative bleeding following tonsillectomy. The trial was double-blind but the method of randomization was not stated. The evaluation of blood loss was graded subjectively, and not quantitated. The study failed to show any beneficial effect of any drug compared to placebo.

Brown (1958) carried out a controlled trial of Adrenosem® in dermabrasion of cheek scars. The quantitation of blood loss was done by weighing the swabs. Dermabrasion of the first cheek in each patient was carried out and then an injection of 2 ml Adrenosem® given. After 30 minutes, the second dermabrasion was done. Of 200 dermabrasion procedures, there was an average calculated reduction of blood loss of 47.9 g of blood per patient, indicating that Adrenosem® was a valuable aid to plastic surgery.

Singhal (1960) carried out a controlled 'double-blind' trial with Adrenoxyl® on 44 cases having removal of sloughs and cutting of skin grafts in burned patients. Blood loss was recorded as the length of time for a donor area to stop bleeding, and by the weighing of swabs. The method of allocation to treatment groups was not stated. No reduction in the amount or duration of blood loss from skin graft donor area was demonstrated.

Perkins (1957) studied 24 patients undergoing surgical dental procedures. The first quadrant of the mouth was operated on, following which Adrenosem® was given. Blood loss was determined by aspiration from the mouth into a glass jar. The blood loss following Adrenosem® was 11.1 ml (mean) less than in the first procedure ($p<0.01$).

Twenty-five male students had ear lobe bleeding time tests either with or without Adrenosem®, 10 mg i.m. injection, one hour previously. The bleeding time shortened significantly from a mean of 107 seconds to 84 seconds.

## Conclusions

The literature suggests that carbazochrome salicylate reduces the bleeding time, by a modest amount, in experimental animals and man.

The majority of controlled studies have not shown a meaningful beneficial clinical effect in surgical situations where the drug has been used most widely. On the other hand, several experienced surgeons have believed strongly that carbazochrome plays an important role in the reduction of postoperative haemorrhage. The challenge is given to these investigators to confirm, in controlled studies, that their beliefs are well founded.

## REFERENCES

BACQ Z.M., CHARLIER R., PHILIPPOT E. and DUNON G. (1949) Arch. int. Physiol. 57, 295.
BRACONIER F., LE BIHAN H. and BEAUDET C. (1943) Arch. int. Pharmacodyn. 69, 181.
BROWN W.S. (1958) Control of bleeding after dermabrasion. Northw. Med. (Seattle) 57, 470.
BURKE D.E., POGRUND R.S. and CLARK W.G. (1960) 'Hemostatic agent in control of bleeding'. Abstract 13th Ann. Meeting of Western Society for Clinical Research, California.
CALNAN J. and INNES F.L.F. (1958) Control of bleeding at operation: a trial of adrenochrome monosemicarbazone (Adrenoxyl). Brit. J. plast. Surg. 11, 87.
DUESBERG J.-P. (1947) Le temps de saignement humain selon la technique de Dishoek et Jongkees. Rev. belg. Path. 18, 333.
DURANTE L.J., MOUTSOS A., AMBROSE R.B., DUNCAN W.Y., FLEMING W., ZINSSER H.H. and PHILLIPS L.L. (1962) Postprostatectomy bleeding: analysis of consequences of control by clotting agents and hypothermia. Ann. Surg. 156, 781.
DYKES E.R. and ANDERSON R. (1961) Carbazochrome salicylate as a systemic hemostatic agent in plastic operations. J. Amer. med. Ass., 177, 716.
FORMAN G.H. and NAYLOR M.N. (1964) Haemostatic properties of adrenochrome monosemicarbazone in dental surgery. Brit. dent. J. 117, 280.
GREEN D.E. and RICHTER D. (1937) Biochem. J. 31, 596.
HAGERTY R.F., ZAVERTNIK J.J. and GRIMSON K.S. (1951) Effect of adrenoxyl on blood loss from surgical wounds. Arch. Surg. 62, 420.
HERVE A. and LECOMTE J. (1949) Action de la semi-carbazone de l'adrénochrome sur les petechies provoquées par le rayonnement X. Arch. int. Pharmacodyn.
HORNE H.W. and SCOTT J.M. (1970) Intrauterine contraceptive devices: A double-blind study. Fertil. and Steril. 21, 230.
KLEMM W.R. and BOLTON G.R. (1967) Comparative evaluation of systemic anticoagulants in dogs. Arzneimittel-Forsch. 17, 1573.
MARCUS A.J. and SPAET T.H. (1958) Ineffectiveness of adrenosem in pulmonary surgery. J. thorac. Surg. 35, 821.
PATEL R.B. (1961) Carbazochrome salicylate in the treatment of pulmonary haemorrhage. J. Indian med. Ass. 36, 327.
PERKINS R.E.L. (1957) A clinical investigation of adrenochrome monosemicarbazone sodium salicylate. Oral Surg. 10, 230.
PREVOST H., CORTEREAU H. and PARROT J.-L. (1947) Elévation de la resistance capillaire sous l'influence du leucodérivé de l'iodadrenochrome et de la monosemicarbazone de l'adrenochrome. C.R. Soc. Biol. (Paris) 141, 1043.
ROSKAM J. and DEROUAUX G. (1944) Arch. int. Pharmacodyn. 69, 348.
RUDDELL J.S. (1958) Adrenochrome monosemicarbazone (adrenoxyl). An interim evaluation of its effect in reducing blood loss. Anaesthesia 13, 269.

SINGHAL G.D. (1960) Failure of adrenoxyl as a haemostatic agent in skin graft donor areas. *Brit. J. plast. Surg.* 12, 362.

SWAN H.T., NUTT A.B., JOWETT G.H., FERGUSON W.J.W. and BLACKBURN E.K. (1961) Monosemicarbazone of adrenochrome (adrenoxyl) and cataract surgery. Effect on capillary resistance and incidence of hyphaema. *Brit. J. Ophthal.* 45, 415.

THAJEB S., KURKCUOGLU M. and McELFRESH A.E. (1959) The value of systemic hemostatic drugs. A 'double-blind' evaluation of agents used to increase coagulation during tonsillectomy and adenoidectomy. *Arch. Otolaryng.* 70, 82.

WHITE N.B., IATRIDIS P.G. and FERGUSON J.H. (1966) Adrenochrome semi-carbazone and lack of *in vivo* activation of Hageman factor. *Amer. J. med. Sci.* 251, 668.

ZWEIFACH B.W. and CHAMBERS R. (1950) Action of hyaluronidase extracts on capillary wall. *Ann. N.Y. Acad. Sci.* 52, 1047.

# Comments on adrenochrome

by G. Derouaux, Liège

(1) The haemostatic properties of adrenochrome were originally linked to an adrenergic mechanism mainly because of the biochemical origin of the compound, i.e. an oxidation product of adrenaline. Early work suggested that adrenochrome could act as a 'promediator' of the activity of adrenergic fibres (Derouaux and Roskam, 1939; Derouaux, 1941). Later work by Bacq and Derouaux (1950), however, showed that it was unlikely that an oxidized form of adrenaline could be converted in the body to the non-oxidized, active form. The same view has been expressed in a later paper dealing with naftazone (Derouaux and Thouverez, 1969).

(2) There is evidence that adrenochrome monosemicarbazone has haemostatic properties in rabbits but only when given prophylactically (Derouaux, 1943).

REFERENCES

BACQ Z.M. and DEROUAUX G. (1950). La semicarbazone de l'adrénochrome. *Sem. Hôp. Paris.* 65, 1.

DEROUAUX G. (1941) Etude du méchanisme de l'action hémostatique de l'adrénaline. *Arch. int. Pharmacodyn.* 66, 202.

DEROUAUX G. (1943). Etude expérimentale de l'action hémostatique de la monoxime et de la monosemicarbazone de l'adrénochrome. *Arch. int. Pharmacodyn.* 69, 142.

DEROUAUX G. and ROSKAM J. (1939) Etude expérimentale de l'action hémostatique de l'adrénochrome. *C.R. Soc. Biol. (Paris)* 131, 830.

DEROUAUX G. and THOUVEREZ J.P. (1969) A propos de l'importance du facteur vasculaire dans l'hémostase. *Coagulation* 2, 193.

# Report on 5-hydroxytryptamine creatinine sulphate: Antemovis®

## Chemical definition and pharmacology

Antemovis® is 2-(5-hydroxy-3-indolyl) ethylamine creatinine sulphate. It is the form of 5-hydroxytryptamine (5HT) available for research and clinical use.

5HT is quickly absorbed after parenteral injection. Given orally, it is rapidly degraded and is therefore ineffective. The metabolism of 5HT varies somewhat from one species to another, but in man it undergoes oxidative deamination by MAO to form 5-hydroxyindoleacetaldehyde. This aldehyde is promptly degraded, mainly by further oxidation to 5-hydroxyindoleacetic acid (5-HIAA) by aldehyde dehydrogenase, but also to a small extent by reduction to the corresponding alcohol, 5-hydroxytryptophol. The three enzymes are present in the liver and various tissues, including the brain. The principal metabolite of 5HT, 5-HIAA, is excreted in the urine (2-10 mg daily by the normal adult). Larger amounts of 5-HIAA are excreted by patients with a malignant carcinoid and after the ingestion of 5HT-containing foods. An amount of 5HT roughly equal to that present in the body is synthesized each day. The discovery of a substance that undergoes substantial, continual synthesis and destruction in the body and that possesses intense and varied pharmacological activities has inevitably resulted in a flood of speculation about its physiological function. It is generally agreed that 5HT plays an important role in nervous transmission. In addition, 5HT is recognized as a precusor metabolite for the pineal hormone melatonin.

Other functions however are less obvious. 5HT stimulates or inhibits a variety of smooth muscles and nerves mainly at the level of the cardiovascular, respiratory and gastrointestinal systems.

5HT has no prominent effect on capillary permeability in any species other than rodents, in which it causes an increase. For further accounts and documentation, the review by Goodman and Gilman (1975) should be consulted.

## Theoretical mode of action as a haemostatic agent

For many years it has been considered that circulating 5HT, which is almost entirely localized in the platelets and is released after their activation (release reaction), aids in effecting haemostasis.

Correl et al. (1952) reported that i.v. injection of 5HT stopped the bleeding of peripheral wounds in rats without affecting the coagulation mechanism. Similar experiments performed by a number of investigators under different experimental conditions led to the suggestion that 5HT is involved in haemostasis as a humoral vasoconstrictor (Correale, 1954; Lecomte et al. 1954; Conti and Ricotti, 1955; Fornaroli and Koller, 1955; Esteve and Laporte, 1957; Stefanini and Magalini, 1956; Baserga and Ballerini, 1956; Djerassi et al., 1958; Bracco and Curti, 1958; Brambel and Murphy, 1959). However, many of the effects described were transient, required the rapid administration of large amounts of 5HT and were accompanied by severe side effects such as dyspnoea, convulsions etc.

Zucker and Borrelli (1955), using a bioassay procedure to measure the concentration of 5HT in platelets, concluded that 5HT accounted for almost all the vasoconstrictive substance(s) in platelets. These authors (1956) also measured the concentration of 5HT in the platelets of patients with various thrombocytopathies and, from the results obtained, suggested that 5HT might be involved in haemostasis in man. During this same period, numerous clinical reports pointed to a haemostatic effectiveness of exogenous 5HT in normal subjects or in patients at risk of haemorrhage (see Maupin, 1960). Some investigators, however, were unable to show any significant effect of exogenous 5HT (administered parenterally) on haemostasis (Miescher, 1955; Stefanini and Magalini, 1956; Jaques et al., 1958). It must be mentioned here that exogenous 5HT is very rapidly taken up by pulmonary endothelial cells and by circulating platelets; any effect of the amine on haemostasis should therefore be mediated through platelets. In view of this property of 5HT, it was essential to evaluate whether platelets deprived of 5HT were haemostatically effective. In this regard, the discovery (Pletscher et al., 1955) that reserpine administration to animals induced the depletion of almost all the 5HT from the platelets (and from the other body depots) was of the greatest importance. Shortly after this, indeed, Shore et al. (1956) determined the bleeding time before and after administration of a single i.v. dose of reserpine to rabbits, rats or guinea pigs. Although the 5HT content of the platelets decreased by more than 90 per cent in the three species, there was no significant alteration in the bleeding time. Haverback *et al.* (1957) administered reserpine i.m. in man daily for one week and found that the platelets were virtually depleted of 5HT. Bleeding time, blood coagulation tests and capillary fragility were not significantly altered.

Goodman and Gilman (1970), commenting upon the role of 5HT in the body's regulation, stated that 'the venerable puzzle of platelet 5HT has not found any solution; the amine does not seem to play any significant role in haemostasis or coagulation'. The same authors (1975), in the latest edition of their textbook, concluded that 'the function of 5HT in platelets is obscure... One view is that platelets serve simply to sequester the 5HT escaping from cells, such as those in the enterochromaffin system'.

Quite recently however, Card and Schiff (1972) reported that five out of seven patients who were taking reserpine (for essential hypertension) at the time of prostatectomy (for benign hyperplasia) bled excessively either during or following operation. There were no abnormalities of clotting time, prothrombin time, partial thromboplastin time, fibrinolytic activity or platelet count in any of the five patients who bled. The authors have postulated that the depression by reserpine of reflex constriction of the veins could render patients treated with reserpine more susceptible to postprostatectomy haemorrhage. The possible role of platelet 5HT in this phenomenon has not been mentioned.

A number of studies performed during the last few years showed that platelet aggregation is accompanied by the generation of a substance called 'rabbit aorta-contracting substance' (Willis, 1974; Vargaftig and Zirinis, 1973). This substance is an intermediate in prostaglandin biosynthesis from arachidonic acid (Gryglewski and Vane, 1972) and might be identical to the potent platelet aggregating compound called 'thromboxane $A_2$' (Hamberg *et al.*, 1975). On a molar basis, it is at least as potent as angiotensin II in causing rabbit aorta to contract (Needleman *et al.*, 1976). The high potency of thromboxane $A_2$, together with its very limited stability at 37°C, has led Needleman *et al.* (1976) to suggest that this substance is a local hormone. Thromboxane $A_2$ generated by adhesive and/or aggregating platelets could produce a profound vasoconstriction largely restricted to the area of the vessel immediately adjacent to the platelet plug. The concept that, when a vessel is injured, the adjacent uninjured vessel contracts only in the presence of a normal platelet plug was clearly established by Zucker (1947).

Drugs such as aspirin or indomethacin that inhibit thromboxane $A_2$ biosynthesis could reduce local vasoconstriction as well as platelet aggregation and thereby prolong the bleeding time (de Gaetano et al., 1975; Needleman et al., 1976).

In conclusion, vasoconstriction related to platelet activation possibly plays a role in the arrest of bleeding. There is no convincing evidence, at present, that 5HT is of major importance in determining the haemostatic effect of platelets. It seems likely that other substances, such as the recently described thromboxane $A_2$, play the major role in this aspect of normal and abnormal haemostasis.

## Clinical efficacy of Antemovis®

All of the clinical studies mentioned under the preceding paragraph and aimed at establishing the haemostatic efficacy of this drug meet the minimal criteria required for a meaningful clinical trial. The possible haemostatic effect of the drug when applied topically, is beyond the scope of the present symposium.

## Side effects

Vertigo, tachycardia and other subjective symptoms of discomfort have been noted in some patients receiving the drug by rapid intravenous injection (see e.g. Greco, 1957).

## Dosage forms and recommended dose (by the manufacturer)

5 mg ampoules (injectable i.m.); 1-2 ampoules every 4-6 hours.

## Conclusions

There is no evidence at present that 5-hydroxytryptamine creatinine sulphate (Antemovis®) is a haemostatic agent in man.

REFERENCES

BASERGA A. and BALLERINI G. (1956) Sérotonine et hémostase spontanée. In *Journées Thérapeutiques de Paris*, pp. 239-247.

BRACCO M. and CURTI P.C. (1958) La 5-ossitriptamina (enteraminaserotonina). *Recenti Progr. Med.* 25, 425.

BRAMBEL Ch.E. and MURPHY D. (1959) Experimental studies with 5-hydroxytryptamine (serotonin) as a hemostyptic agent following traumatic injury after irradiation in white rats. *Thrombos. Diathes. haemorrh (Stuttg.)* 3, 354.

CARD D.J. and SCHIFF M.Jr. (1972) Possible role of reserpine in postprostatectomy hemorrhage. *J. Urol. (Baltimore)* 107, 97.

CONTI U. and RICOTTI G.F. (1955) L'azione della 5-ossitriptamina sulle emorragie parenchimali (a nappo). *Farmaco, Ed. sci.* 10, 637.

CORREALE P. (1954) Azione dell'enteramina (5-idrossi-triptamina) sulla pressione sistemica e sull' emostasi nel ratto. *Arch. int. Pharmacodyn.* 97, 106.

CORRELL J.T., LYTH L.F., LONG S. and VANDERPOEL J.C. (1952) Some physiological responses to 5-hydroxytryptamine creatinine sulfate. *Amer. J. Physiol.* 169, 537.

DE GAETANO G., DONATI M.B. and GARATTINI S. (1975) Drugs affecting platelet function tests. Their effects on haemostasis and surgical bleeding. *Thrombos. Diathes. haemorrh. (Stuttg.)* 34, 285.

DJERASSI I., KLEIN E., FARBER S. and PALMER D. (1958) Effects of 5-hydroxytryptamine on some aspects of the hemorrhagic state in radiation-induced thrombocytopenia. *Proc. Soc. Exp. Biol. (N.Y.)* 97, 552.

ESTEVE A. and LAPORTE J. (1957) L'action de certains antihémorragiques sur le prolongement du temps de saignement provoqués par quelques médicaments. *Thérapie* 12, 510.

FORNAROLI P. and KOLLER M. (1955) Prove sperimentali sull-azione emostatica della 5-ossitriptamina nell'animale normale. *Farmaco, Ed. sci.* 10, 91.

GOODMAN L.S. and GILMAN A. eds. (1970) *The Pharmacological Basis of Therapeutics*, 4th ed., pp. 645-662, MacMillan, New York.

GOODMAN L.S. and GILMAN A. eds. (1975) *The Pharmacological Basis of Therapeutics*, 5th ed., pp. 613-629, MacMillan, New York.

GRECO A.S. (1957) Impiego del solfato doppio di 5-ossitriptamina e creatinina (Antemovis) in soggetti con emostasi normale operati di tonsillectomia. *Minerva otorinolaring.* 7, 3.

GRYGLEWSKI R. and VANE J.R. (1972) The generation from arachidonic acid of rabbit aorta contracting substance (RCS) by a microsomal enzyme preparation which also generates prostaglandins. *Brit. J. Pharmacol.* 46, 449.

HAMBERG M., SVENSSON J. and SAMUELSSON B. (1975) Thromboxanes: A new group of biologically active compounds derived from prostaglandin endoperoxides. *Proc. Natl. Acad. Sci. (Wash.)* 72, 2994.

HAVERBACK B.J., DUTCHER T.F., SHORE P.A., TOMICH E.G., TERRY L.L. and BRODIE B.B. (1957) Serotonin changes in platelets and brain induced by small daily doses of reserpine - lack of effect of depletion of platelet serotonin on hemostatic mechanisms. *New Engl. J. Med.* 256, 343.

JACQUES L.B., FISHER L.M. and ASHWIN J. (1958) Platelet serotonin as a factor in hemostasis. (Abstract). 7th Congress Intern. Soc. Transfusion, Rome.

LECOMTE J., BOUNAMEAUX Y., FISCHER P. and OSTERRIETH P. (1954) Action de la 5-hydroxytryptamine sur le temps de saignement moyen chez le lapin. *Arch. int. Pharmacodyn. Ther.* 97, 389.

MAUPIN B. (1960) La sérotonine. Dosage. Métabolisme. Pharmacologie. Quelques aspects biologiques. *Biol. méd. (Paris)* 49, 75.

MIESCHER P. (1955) Discussion to paper of Baserga A. and Ballerini G. La 5-hydroxytryptamine dans la thérapie des hémorragies thrombocytopeniques. *Schweiz. med. Wschr.* 85, 914.

NEEDLEMAN P., MONCADA S., BUNTING S., VANE J.R., HAMBERG M. and SAMUELSSON B. (1976) Identification of an enzyme in platelet microsomes which generates thromboxane $A_2$ from prostaglandin endoperoxides. *Nature (Lond.)* 261, 558.

PLETSCHER A., SHORE P.A. and BRODIE B.B. (1955) Serotonin release as a possible mechanism of reserpine action. *Science* 122, 374.

SHORE P.A., PLETSCHER A., TOMICH E.G., KUNTZMAN R. and BRODIE B.B. (1956) Release of blood platelet serotonin by reserpine and lack of effect on bleeding time. *J. Pharmacol. exp. Ther.* 117, 232.

STEFANINI M. and MAGALINI S.I. (1956) Evaluation of the hemostatic properties of synthetic serotonin. *Arch. intern. Med.* 98, 23.

VARGAFTIG B.B. and ZIRINIS P. (1973) Platelet aggregation induced by arachidonic acid is accompanied by release of potential inflammatory mediators distinct from $PGE_2$ and $PGF_2\alpha$. *Nature (New Biol.)* 244, 114.

WILLIS A.L. (1974) An enzymatic mechanism for the antithrombotic and antihemostatic actions of aspirin. *Science* 183, 325.

ZUCKER M.B. (1947) Platelet agglutination and vasoconstriction as factors in spontaneous hemostasis in normal, thrombocytopenic, heparinized and hypoprothrombinemic rats. *Amer. J. Physiol.* 148, 275.

ZUCKER M.B. and BORRELLI J. (1955) Quantity, assay, and release of serotonin in human platelets. *J. appl. Physiol.* 7, 425.

ZUCKER M.B. and BORRELLI J. (1956) Concentration of serotonin in serum, in thrombocytopathia, pseudohemophilia and thrombocytosis. *Amer. J. clin. Path.* 26, 13.

# Report on a preparation of conjugated oestrogens[1]: Premarin®

## Chemical composition.

Naturally occuring conjugated oestrogens prepared from pregnant mares' urine.

## Presentation.

(1) Freeze dried powder with sterile diluent for intravenous or intramuscular injection.
(2) Tablets for oral administration.

## Mode of action.

Only speculation on modes of action has been possible. It has been proposed that Premarin® may act by the following mechanisms.
(1) By altering the nature of the 'ground substance' of connective tissue. Within 15 minutes to 3 hours of intravenous injection of Premarin® into man or experimental animals, alterations in the connective tissue around small blood vessels and in arteriole walls have been reported; there has been:
(a) an increase in the quantity of acid mucopolysaccharide
(b) an increase in the degree of polymerization of mucopolysaccharide
(c) an increase in the number and activity of mast cells.

The first two changes are thought to alter the gel/sol equilibrium in the tissues in favour of the gel phase (Schiff and Burn, 1961). Alteration in the hyaluronidase-induced cutaneous weal after administration of Premarin® and a rise in the serum level of a non-specific hyaluronidase inhibitor

1. Other preparations of conjugated oestrogens: Dagynil®, Equigyne®, Presomen®.

were also reported as evidence for an effect on ground substance (Wayne *et al.*, 1964); the reduced pulmonary diffusing capacity after Premarin® administration was likewise held to indicate such an effect (Pecora *et al.*, 1963).

(2) Changes in the blood haemostatic mechanism have been proposed as a means by which a haemostatic effect is attained. A sharp rise in factor V levels with an increase in prothrombin activity was reported after injection of Premarin® into dogs (Johnson, 1957) and a small decrease in antithrombin activity was also recorded. No change or only trivial alteration in the haemostatic parameters of humans after injection of Premarin® has been reported (Borchgrevink *et al.*, 1960; McGovern *et al.*, 1961; Wayne *et al.*, 1964); prolonged oral administration of Premarin® does alter factor VII and factor X activity however (Poller *et al.*, 1977). Reduced antithrombin III levels after Premarin® ingestion have been recorded in humans (von Kaulla *et al.*, 1975). Increased euglobulin caseinolytic activity (Nagayama *et al.*, 1965) but, in contrast, no change in the euglobulin lysis time (von Kaulla *et al.*, 1975) have been reported.

Platelet aggregation by ADP and noradrenaline was enhanced by oral Premarin® (Elkeles *et al.*, 1968) but no change in platelet adhesiveness was observed after oral (Elkeles *et al.*, 1968) or intravenous administration (Borchgrevink *et al.*, 1960). No alteration in the bleeding time has been reported (Borchgrevink *et al.*, 1960; Wayne *et al.*, 1964).

**Animal and human pharmacology.**

Few data are available. The absence of an easily measurable effect on the haemostatic mechanism renders this difficult. The alterations noted in connective tissue in humans were evident within 15 minutes (Schiff and Burn, 1961). The alterations noted in the coagulation system of dogs were evident within 15 minutes and maximal between 30 and 150 minutes after injection of Premarin® (Johnson, 1957).

**Clinical efficacy in patients with a bleeding disorder.**

Accounts have appeared of the apparent efficacy of various oestrogen preparations in the treatment of a variety of bleeding disorders such as hereditary haemorrhagic telangiectasia (Koch *et al.*, 1952) and haemophilia (Whittington, 1956). A description of the use of Premarin® in the management of a wide range of bleeding symptoms in patients maintained on long term oral anticoagulant drugs of the coumarin series has also appeared (Roberts, 1961); the precise role of Premarin® in the control of bleeding is difficult to ascertain as anticoagulant drugs were usually discontinued and, occasionally, vitamin K analogues were administered in addition. No controlled study of the effect of Premarin® on bleeding symptoms in patients with haemorrhagic disorders has appeared.

## Clinical efficacy in patients without a bleeding disorder.

Numerous descriptions of the control by Premarin® of many different bleeding symptoms in patients not known to have a bleeding disorder have been recorded (Jacobson, 1954; Menger, 1955; Whittington, 1956; Popper, 1960; Withers, 1960; Narang, 1962; Roberts, 1961; Fabrykant *et al.*, 1964). In the majority of studies which have been controlled and in which an attempt has been made to quantify blood loss, and in almost all studies conducted on a double blind basis no significant effect of Premarin® in reducing blood loss has been demonstrated (Borchgrevinck *et al.*, 1960; Cooner and Burros, 1960; McDonough and Mulla, 1961; Thajeb *et al.*, 1959; McGovern *et al.*, 1961; Verstraete *et al.*, 1968). In one blind trial, however, use of Premarin® was associated with significant reduction of blood loss during cardiac surgery (Ambrus *et al.*, 1971).

## Side effects.

Headache and nausea have been recorded after intravenous injection (Jacobson, 1954) and slow injection is advised to avoid flushing. Absence of side effects has been reported in some studies (Menger, 1955; Borchgrevink *et al.*, 1960). As recommendations for control of bleeding involve intravenous administration on a limited number of occasions, the usual side effects associated with oestrogens should be avoided. The only recommended contraindication is gross hepatic disease.

## Recommended dose.

25 mg given slowly intravenously or intramuscularly is recommended as the therapy for 'spontaneous capillary bleeding'. A response is expected within 60 minutes and the dose may be repeated. A similar dose is recommended as prophylaxis prior to surgery.

## Conclusions.

This review is concerned primarily with the efficacy of Premarin® as a haemostatic agent. As such it does not impinge on the suggested use of the material in other fields such as replacement therapy; indeed in literature discussing the use of Premarin® orally as replacement therapy the makers point out that its use is not associated with altered platelet behaviour or change in the clotting profile.

In spite, therefore, of case descriptions associating the intravenous administration of Premarin® with dramatic cessation of spontaneous and traumatic bleeding, most controlled studies have failed to indicate that it is useful in the control of surgical bleeding. Its use in the control of spontaneous bleeding such as epistaxis and haemoptysis has not been rigorously examined; in one small double-blind trial of its effects on severe epistaxis Premarin® was not superior to a placebo (Borchgrevink et al., 1960).

### REFERENCES

AMBRUS J.L., SCHIMERT G., LAJOS T.Z., AMBRUS C.M., MINK I.B., LASSMANN H.B., MOORE R.H. and MELZER J. (1971) Effect of antifibrinolytic agents and estrogens on blood loss and blood coagulation factors during open heart surgery. J. Med. 2, 65.

BORCHGREVINK C.F., ANDERSEN R., HALL J., HATTELAND K. and URSIN-HOLM A. (1960) 'Premarin' as a haemostatic agent: failure to demonstrate any laboratory or clinical effect. Brit. med. J. ii, 1645.

COONER W.H. and BURROS H.M. (1960) Clinical evaluation of effect of Premarin on bleeding during and following prostatic surgery. J. Urol. (Baltimore) 83, 64.

ELKELES R.S., HAMPTON J.R. and MITCHELL J.R.A. (1968) Effect of oestrogens on human platelet behaviour. Lancet ii, 315.

FABRYKANT M., GELFAND M.L. and ROSENBERG A.S. (1964) Further experience with anabolic steroids in diabetic retinopathy. Amer. J. med. Sci. 248, 304.

JACOBSON P. (1954) Spontaneous hemorrhage. Arch. Otolaryng. 59, 523.

JOHNSON J.F. (1957) Changes in plasma prothrombin, Ac-globulin, and antithrombin concentration following intravenous administration of estrogens. Proc. Soc. exp. Biol. Med. 94, 92.

KOCH H.J., ESCHER G.C. and LEWIS J.S. (1952) Hormonal management of hereditary haemorrhagic telangiectasia. *J. Amer. med. Ass.* 149, 1376.

McDONOUGH J.J. and MULLA N. (1961) Blood loss in vaginal operations and the use of preoperation intravenous estrogen. *Amer. J. Obstet. Gynec.* 82, 565.

McGOVERN J.J., BUNKER J.P., GOLDSTEIN R. and ESTES J.W. (1961) Effect of conjugated estrogens on the coagulation mechanism. *J. Amer. med. Ass.* 175, 1011.

MENGER H.C. (1955) Estrogen given parenterally to control epistaxis and haemorrhage after adenoidectomy. *J. Amer. med. Ass.* 159, 546.

NAGAYAMA M., MAKI M., KIKUCHI I., KANBE K., SASAKI K. and SASAKI K. (1965) Effect of estrogens on blood clotting and plasmin systems. *Tohoku J. exp. Med.* 86, 219.

NARANG R.K. (1962) Role of sodium estrone sulfate (Premarin®) in haemoptysis. *Amer. Rev. resp. Dis.* 85, 436.

PECORA L.J., PUTNAM L.R. and BAUM G.L. (1963) Effects of intravenous estrogens on pulmonary diffusing capacity. *Amer. J. med. Sci.* 246, 48.

POLLER L., THOMSON J.M. and COOPE J. (1977) Conjugated equine oestrogens and blood clotting: a follow-up report. *Brit. med. J.* i, 935.

POPPER J. (1960) Use of Premarin iv in hemoptysis. *Dis. Chest* 37, 659.

ROBERTS H.R. (1961) Oral and intravenous estrogens in the treatment and prevention of bleeding associated with long term anticoagulant therapy. *J. Amer. Geriat. Soc.* 9, 184.

SCHIFF M. and BURN H.F. (1961) The effect of intravenous oestrogens on ground substance. *Arch. Otolaryng.* 73, 44.

THAJEB S., KURKCUOGLU M. and McELFRESH A.E. (1959) Value of systemic hemostatic drugs: double blind evaluation of agents used to increase coagulation during tonsillectomy and adenoidectomy. *Arch. Otolaryng.* 70, 72.

VERSTRAETE M., VERMYLEN J. and TYBERGHEIN J. (1968) Double blind evaluation of the haemostatic effect of adrenochrome monosemicarbazone; conjugated oestrogens and epsilon aminocaproic acid after adenotonsillectomy. *Acta haemat. (Basel)* 40, 154.

VON KAULLA E., DROEGEMUELLER W., and VON KAULLA K.N. (1975) Conjugated estrogens and hypercoagulability. *Amer. J. Obstet. Gynec.* 122, 688.

WAYNE L., GLUECK H.I., BRODINE C. and COOTS M. (1964) Effect of intravenous estrogen on an inhibitor of hyaluronidase and on clotting factors in blood. *Proc. Soc. exp. Biol. (N.Y.)* 116, 85.

WITHERS B.T. (1960) Facility in tonsilloadenoidectomy management. Conclusions from 2,400 consecutive cases. *Arch. Otolaryng.* 72, 183.

WHITTINGTON P.B. (1956) Control of bleeding with intravenous estrogens. *J. Amer. dent. Ass.* 53, 595.

# Comments by the manufacturer of Premarin®

## by M. Gahwyler, Ayerst International, New York

It is a very well known fact that to date medical science is missing easy and subjective techniques of measuring exact blood loss, both in animal and human clinical research. Thus the evaluation of any haemostatic agent is very difficult to assess, especially in some surgical procedures during which the blood loss is *ex-equo* minimal. In this present form, the review appears to deny the prophylactic or therapeutic usefulness of Premarin® Parenteral in the different fields of surgery. This is, however, based only on an incomplete bibliography related to this subject.

In the past few years there have been many reports on the use of water-soluble oestrogens to reduce haemorrhage in various clinical fields. The oestrogens have been used to reduce capillary bleeding both spontaneous and surgically induced; in epistaxis and following tonsillectomy, in traumatic hyphaemia, following prostatectomies and in haemoptysis and post-operative bleeding following open-heart surgery.

The mode of action of the water-soluble oestrogens is not fully understood, although they are known to shorten bleeding time.

The following facts about the action of the drug on clotting and bleeding have been reported and may be summarized under four headings:
(1) Influence on blood clotting factors
(2) Influence on connective tissue
(3) Influence on blood platelets
(4) Influence on fibrinolysis

### Influence on blood clotting factors

Johnson (1957) showed that following injection of Premarin®, there was an elevation in the levels of prothrombin and factor V and reduction in the antithrombin activity of the plasma.

The experiments were done on individuals with normal clotting mechanisms, so that these changes cannot explain the haemostatic effect of Premarin®, as an elevation of a factor present in normal amounts is not expected to improve the overall clotting mechanism (Schiff and Burn, 1961; Wayne et al., 1964).

### Influence on connective tissue

It has been shown that conjugated oestrogens increase the content of mucopolysaccharides in connective tissue, especially that of hyaluronic acid (Ulutin, 1969).

The mode of action of Premarin® is to increase the hyaluronidase inhibitor of the serum, and thus decrease hyaluronidase activity. This causes an increase in the mucopolysaccharide content of the connective tissue, lengthens the polymers of the molecules, and shifts the sol-gel equilibrium to the gel side.

This effect is most pronounced in the basal membrane of the small vessels and in the perivascular tissue. Thus there is a vascular and perivascular decrease in permeability, leading to reduction of capillary bleeding. This factor is probably the most significant in the clinical reduction of capillary bleeding.

### Influence on platelets

Premarin® does not increase the number of platelets but has been shown to increase their adhesiveness. The mechanism of this action is unclear but it may be related to the fact that the platelet produces and contains mucopolysaccharides, and a similar effect to that described above may also apply (Elkeles, 1968).

### Influence on fibrinolysis

Schersten (1958) showed that Premarin® caused an increase in the level of fibrinogen by inhibition of fibrinolysis. The importance of this in capillary bleeding is still unclear.

There is still growing interest, both in basic research and on the clinical usefulness of Premarin® Parenteral in different fields of surgical approaches, by very well known representatives in the medical profession.

Let me bring to your attention the results obtained by Dr. Tsur, from the Plastic Surgery Department of Montefiore Hospital in New York, which were recently presented at the Research Council in Denver, Colorado. The author used very sophisticated parameters to measure the blood loss and demonstrated that there is a statistically significant reduction in surgically-induced bleeding in rats following the injection of Premarin® Parenteral. A mean value of 44% reduction of blood loss was measured. In addition to this, Dr. Bornstein, Chairman of the Chaim Hospital and Medical Center in Tel-Hashomer, Israel, and President of the International Society of Plastic Surgeons, has been involved in clinical research with Premarin® Parenteral since 1972, and has obtained dramatic modification of blood loss using Premarin® Parenteral.

Finally, the report never mentions the usefulness of Premarin® Parenteral in cases of dysfunctional uterine bleeding (abnormal uterine bleeding due to hormonal imbalance in the absence of organic causes) where it is recognized by many clinicians as a drug of choice. This indication is completely omitted in this review.

Considering the above points of view, would it not be appropriate to include these facts in the final conclusion of the report, as these represent the most recent data, and would also acknowledge controlled double-blind clinical research in progress.

REFERENCES

AMBRUS J.L., SCHIMERT G., LAJOS T.Z., AMBRUS C.M., MINK I.B., LASSMAN H.B., MOORE R.H. and MELZER J. (1971) Effect of antifibrinolytic agents and estrogens on blood loss and blood coagulation factors during open heart surgery. *J. Med.* 2, 65.

ELKELES R.S., HAMPTON J.R. and MICHELL J.R.A. (1968) Effect of oestrogens on human platelet behaviour. *Lancet* ii, 315.

JOHNSON J.F. (1957) Changes in plasma prothrombin, Ac-globulin and antithrombin concentration following intravenous administration of estrogens. *Proc. Soc. exp. Biol. (N.Y.)* 94, 92.

SCHERSTEN B. (1958) On haemostatics with particular reference to their clinical use. *Suom. Laak.* 13, 855.

SCHIFF M. and BURN H.F. (1961) The effect of intravenous oestrogens on ground substance. *Arch. Otolaryng.* 73, 44.

ULUTIN O.N. (1969) Sex hormones and blood coagulation. In: *Recent Advances in Blood Coagulation.* (Poller L., ed.), pp. 215-228, Churchill, London.

WAYNE L., GLUECK H.I., BRODINE C. and COOTS M. (1964) Effect of intravenous estrogen on an inhibitor of hyaluronidase and on clotting factors in blood. *Proc. Soc. exp. Biol. (N.Y.)* 116, 85.

# Report on a preparation of oestriol succinate[1]: Styptanon®

Oestriol disodium succinate was introduced as a haemostatic agent by Organon about twelve years ago. In the Netherlands it is still sold under what our American colleagues call the 'grandfather clause', in other words, it counts as an old drug which has not yet been evaluated for efficacy and safety by the Netherlands Committee for the Evalution of Medicines. In current promotional literature the manufacturer recommends that the product be administered parenterally in cases of capillary bleeding during or after surgical operations, and in parenchymal bleeding. It is also recommended for 'conditions associated with derangement of permeability and fragility of the capillaries'. Doses of 20 mg are injected once or twice; they can be given either intravenously or intramuscularly.

## Chemical composition

Oestriol is of course a natural oestrogen, normally present in the female organism. It has been stated to be an 'impeded oestrogen' in that hormonal doses do not exhibit the full spectrum of oestrogenic activity, but this may reflect the fact that it is a relatively weak oestrogen and that not all receptors are equally sensitive to oestrogenic activity.

The succinate does not appear to differ in its hormonal properties from the parent substance, though it may be pharmacokinetically slightly different (van der Vies, 1965).

## Mode of action

The concept that oestrogens might be of value as haemostyptic agents is quite an old one.

Some pointers to it were available as early as 1931. De Silva, Heimberg

1. Other preparations of oestriol succinate: Ovestin®.

and Zuckermann all worked on the problem during the years which followed. Since some of the first evidence related to the successful treatment of menorrhagia, it was obviously tempting to regard the effect as one specific to the endometrium, as one would expect with oestrogens; however, some evidence was obtained that other types of haemorrhage too might react. The fact that haemophilia is a more common cause of bleeding in men than in women was readily attributed to the level of circulating oestrogens in women. In 1941, Jacobson in the United States concluded that there was a correlation between spontaneous epistaxis and oestrogen levels, and he used conjugated oestrogens to treat the condition. Other clinicians used these products to reduce retinal bleeding, to counter blood loss in surgery, and to alleviate purpura.

Most of the early work was performed with conjugated oestrogens, but it was entirely logical for a manufacturer producing oestriol to look into the possibility of using this substance for the same purpose, since one would hope to attain a haemostatic effect disocciated from unwanted endocrine activity; by using the sodium salt of the succinate it would be possible to administer the substance intravenously when needed to attain a rapid effect.

The work with oestriol, in particular, threw some light on the way in which oestrogens might be expected to act on bleeding.

Clinical impressions that oestrogens were capable of relieving haemorrhagic diatheses of various origin suggested that investigation should be directed to their effects on the vascular wall. Work both in human subjects and animals led to the conclusion that oestriol succinate had three clinical effects; it appeared to improve reduced capillary resistance, to decrease capillary fragility and to normalize increased capillary permeability. Histochemically, changes in the pericapillary ground substance and the periarteriolar connective tissue were found (Staubesand et al., 1963, 1966; Poliwoda, 1965); there appeared to be an increase in the proportion of acid mucopolysaccharides. At the same time, various workers looked into the possibility of an effect on the clotting and fibrinolytic system. No effects on the usual parameters of blood clotting or on clotting factors were reported, but there was an improvement in the pathologically decreased platelet adhesion in such conditions as von Willebrand's disease (Winckelmann and Köhler, 1964), the latter perhaps due to an effect on the wall rather than on the platelets themselves.

Almost all this work dates from the mid sixties; since then much more work has been done with oestrogens and their effects on blood clotting and fibrinolysis, but the newer work relates mostly to the stronger oestrogens used in oral contraceptives, and it does not necessarily hold good for oestriol succinate.

## Animal and human pharmacology

In view of the hypothesis that the effect was mostly on the vascular wall, the animal pharmacological models were directed mainly to this question.

Bonta and his staff developed a model based on the ability of the venom of the *Naja-Naja* snake to damage the vessel wall (Bonta *et al.*, 1965). In canine heart-lung preparations, for example, local application of the venom onto the pulmonary surface produced reproducible local haemorrhages. If oestriol succinate was either applied locally or added to the circulating blood, the haemorrhages appeared later and were less severe. Another model involved intact mice, which received an intra-thoracic dose of venom, sufficient to induce fatal pulmorary bleeding; if the oestrogen was given systemically or locally in advance, it reduced the degree of haemorrhage and it prolonged survival time (Bonta *et al.*, 1965). One must however add that in the light of recent work one can conclude that snake-venom studies detect anti-inflammatory rather than anti-haemorrhagic activity (Bonta and Vargaftig, 1976).

The same group found that in mice, oestriol succinate given intraven-ously was able to prevent pulmonary haemorrhages induced by sudden decompression suggesting that the vessel walls were being rendered more resistent to injury (Bonta and de Vos, 1962).

Finally, these workers found oestriol succinate to be capable of inhibiting the development of oedema in the rat paw induced by such agents as histamine, serotonin and kaolin (de Vos and Bonta, 1965). This again would, however, seem to point to anti-inflammatory activity.

A more general cautionary point which should be noted at this stage is that the dosages employed in the animal experiments were generally such that one can hardly extrapolate the findings to man. In the decompres-sion test, for example, 2 x 200 mg/kg was given i.v., some 400-800 times the human dose per unit weight.

The same discrepancy is found in some animal work from other groups e.g. Kronberger (1965) who studied bleeding in rabbits after standardised laceration but gave these small animals the full human dose. However in the heart-lung test it was shown that an effect was obtained with blood concentrations of 5-10 µg/ml, and these levels are much more closely comparable to what one might briefly attain in man after a dose of 40 mg, although there is not much exact pharmacokinetic data on the preparation.

## Clinical efficacy

There are some forty clinical reports bearing on Styptanon®, but as with many older drugs the work was not performed according to the standards likely to be applied at the present day.

The majority of papers relate to large and very mixed series of patients. Pierer, for example (1964) reports that of 97 cases, 82 reacted favourably to Styptanon®. His report however relates to therapeutic use in 15 different diagnoses and to prophylactic pre-operative use in 23 cases; most of his material concerns patients with disorders of the gastrointestinal and urinary tract, including carcinomas, ulcers and varices, and one would expect the efficacy of a product acting on the capillary wall to differ quite substantially in these different diagnostic groups.

A quite different but again very heterogeneous series is that described by Poliwoda and his colleagues in 1963; some 281 cases are summarised, with a favourable reaction in the majority, but the conditions range from pulmonary bleeding with bronchiectasis to eight different disorders with secondary thrombocytopenia.

There are various studies with control groups, but apparently none in which a double-blind approach or a proper quantification of blood loss has been adopted, unless the very limited study by Kranzl and Richter (1969) in which only 5 surgical patients were studied with erythrocyte-labelling is considered.

There is also a double-blind study with an oral version of the product (Ohly, 1965) but the results are virtually negative and this form does not appear to have been further developed.

Alongside the many positive clinical impressions there are also negative reports. Bosseckert and Remde (1965) for example saw no clinical or pharmacodynamic effect at all when oestriol succinate was given for up to 20 days in the recommended doses to patients with bleeding of vascular or coagulopathic origin.

## Side effects

The literature does not report any unexpected side effects at all at the recommended doses, but as one would anticipate it is pointed out that if treatment with these dose levels – 20 mg or 40 mg on each occasion – is continued for a long period of time, effects on the mammae and menstrual cycle may occur, since these are substantially higher than the doses of oestriol used to treat vaginal and menopausal complaints.

## Conclusions

The animal pharmacology and some of the clinical pharmacology quite clearly point to the fact that oestrogens do have effects on the vascular wall; the effects are such that one could envisage their being exploited clinically. The clinical material available does not however meet the criteria listed by the organisers of this meeting, a point on which the manufacturers appear to agree. This is unfortunate, because one is dealing here with a rather innocuous natural substance, which might in well-defined conditions be of use as a haemostatic agent. One would, for example, like to follow up some of the older pointers to a correlation between bleeding and oestrogen deficiency; it might be that oestrogens have a specific role to play in preventing or arresting bleeding in oestrogen-deficient subjects. The literature available does not differentiate sufficiently clearly between the response which might be obtained in different types of vascular or haematological disorder. Finally, the extent to which the effects of this oestrogen on clotting, platelet adhesion and fibrinolysis provide sufficient grounds for certain indications (or warnings) must be further investigated.

Much of what has been said here appears to apply equally to conjugated oestrogens, although the literature is less readily accessible. In 1969, at the end of the period during which these products were being actively studied as haemostatics, the Medical Letter reviewed the clinical literature on Premarin®. It concluded that 'there is no acceptable evidence that Premarin® can prevent or control spontaneous capillary bleeding, gastrointestinal bleeding, hemoptysis or bleeding associated with surgery'. It would thus appear that the same desiderata for further study which have been listed for Styptanon® apply to this product, the effects of which are likely to be very similar.

REFERENCES

ANON (1969) Conjugated Estrogens (Premarin) for spontaneous and surgical bleeding. *Medical Letter* 11, 53.

BONTA I. L. and VARGAFTIG B. B. (1976) Cobra venom induced pulmonary vessel lesion; an unconventional model of acute inflammation. *Bull. Inst. Pasteur* 74, 131.

BONTA I. L. and VOS C. J. DE (1962) Antihaemorrhagic and permeability-inhibitor effect of estriol and estriol-16, 17 disodium succinate in animal experiments. Paper read during II Intern-Gespräch über Angiologie, Darmstadt, 24-28 Oct.

BONTA I.L., VOS G.J. DE, and DELVER A. (1965) Inhibitory effects of estriol-16, 17-disodium succinate on local haemorrhages induced by snake venom in canine heart-lung preparations. *Acta Endocr. (Kbh.)* 48, 137.

BOSSECKERT H. and REMDE W. (1965) Klinische Untersuchungen zur hämostyptischen Wirkung von Oestriol. *Folia Haemat*, (Lpz.) 84, 234.

JACOBSON P. (1941) *Virginia med. Mth.* 68, 37.

KRANZL B. and RICHTER H. (1969) Messungen des Blutverlustes bei Kieferchirurgischen Operationen unter Wirkung von Oestriolsuccinat. *Z. Stomat.* 66, 96.

KRONBERGER L. (1965) Uber den hämostyptischen Effekt des Ostriolsuccinates. *Wien. klin. Wschr.* 77, 881.

OHLY A. (1965) *Uber den Einfluss von Ostriolsuccinat auf Mikrohänaturien und Blutungszwischenfälle bei Patienten under Langzeit-Antikoagulantien Therapie.* Thesis, University of Munich.

PIERER H. (1964) Ergebnisse einer kritischen Klinischen Prüfung der hämostyptischen Wirkung von Ostriolsuccinat. *Med. Klin.* 59, 1876.

POLIWODA H. (1965) Die medikamentöse Therapie von Blutungen unter Berucksichtigung ihrer Ätiologie und Pathogenese. *Landarzt* 41, 1468.

POLIWODA H., SCHMIDT-MATTHIESEN H. and BARTHELS M. (1963) Klinische Erfahrungen mit Ostriolsuccinat bei der Behandlung hämorrhagischer Diathesen in der inneren Medizin, Geburtshilfe und Gynäkologie. *Schweiz. med. Wschr.* 93, 1568.

STAUBESAND J., SCHMIDT-MATTHIESEN H. and POLIWODA H. (1963) Elektronmikroskopische und histochemische Befunde zum Problem des sogenannten Gefässfaktors gewisser haemorrhagischer Diathesen. (Electron-Microscopic and Histochemical Findings on the so called Vascular-Factor by certain Forms of Haemorrhagic Diathesis). *Dtsch. med. Wschr.* 2 (6), 7.

STAUBESAND J., SCHMIDT-MATTHIESEN H. and POLIWODA H. (1966) Elektronenmikroskopische und histochemische Befunde zum Problem des sog. Gefässfaktors bei hämorrhagischen Diathesen. *Klin. Wschr.* 44, 547.

VIES J. VAN DER (1965) Fate of Oestriol-16, 17 dihemisuccinate after oral administration to rats. *Acta Endocr.* (Kbh.) 48, 630.

VOS C.J. DE and BONTA I.L. (1965) Inhibitory effect of estriol-16, 17-disodium succinate in various kinds of rat paw edema. *Acta physiol. pharmacol. neerl.* 13.

WINCKELMANN G. and KOHLER H. (1964) Die Beeinflussung der Plättchenadhäsivität beim v. Willebrand-Jürgens-Syndrom durch Oestriolsuccinat. *Klin. Wschr.* 42, 1098.

# Comments by the manufacturer of Styptanon®

**by T. Vossenaar, Organon International BV, Oss (Holland)**

The appreciation by the expert clearly recognizes the influence of oestrogens on the vascular wall. However, it is stated that the clinical proof is not according to the standards required in 1977.

This touches upon a problem that is of a far more general nature than related to Styptanon® only. Through the developments in clinical pharmacology and the methodology of clinical investigation as well as through the increased requirements of registration authorities a situation has arisen whereby nearly all clinical trials performed more than ± 10 years ago can be considered to be more or less obsolete. If this development continues, it may well be that in due time the same can be said for investigations that we are performing now and that according to our beliefs are in conformity with present standards. Therefore, I consider it justified, when looking at old preparations, to make a distinction between on the one hand those compounds where a basic rationale is present and where clinical experience in actual practice over many years has shown them to be effective as well as devoid of side-effects, and on the other hand those compounds where the basic research is insufficient, where efficacy is doubtful and where side-effects are present to such a degree that they must give rise to caution. I take the view that for the first category of drugs it is not justified to spend research money and to use clinical facilities for further work and that it is better to concentrate on those products where additional work is clearly required.

In my opinion Styptanon® belongs to the group of preparations where a sound theoretical basis and 12 years of satisfactory clinical experience are present. This implies that further clinical work at this moment is in my opinion, also in relation to priorities to be made, not warranted.

# Report on a preparation of snake venom (from Bothrops jararaca)[1]: Botropase®

## Chemical definition

Botropase® is a coagulant fraction having a thrombin-like activity which is extracted from the venom of *Bothrops jararaca.*

## Mode of action

The thrombin-like enzyme in Botropase® converts fibrinogen to fibrin (des A-fibrin) by the removal of fibrinopeptide A only (Blombäck *et al.*, 1957; Dinelli *et al.*, 1959; Stocker and Straub, 1970). This enzyme is not inhibited by heparin or the antithrombin system in human plasma (de Nicola *et al.*, 1969). The interaction of Botropase® with fibrinogen *in vivo* has been demonstrated (Lampugnani and Cultrera, 1970). Low levels of this agent can be expected to introduce low grade diffuse intravascular coagulation (DIC) associated with the formation of soluble fibrin monomer complexes (SFMC). Thus blood in this hypercoagulable state would be expected to clot more readily. While the literature does not stress that Botropase® contains a thromboplastin-like activity, such an activity seems to be evident in the presence of platelets (de Nicola *et al.*, 1969; Gibelli and Giarola, 1973). The drug might thus be expected to generate thrombin which would be neutralised by the plasma antithrombin system. Figure 1 schematically outlines these mechanisms of action of Botropase®.

## Animal and human pharmacology

Toxicity studies (Leroy, 1965; de Nicola, personal communication, 1976) suggest that guinea pigs and pigeons suffered no visible discomfort

1. Similar preparation: Ophidiase®.

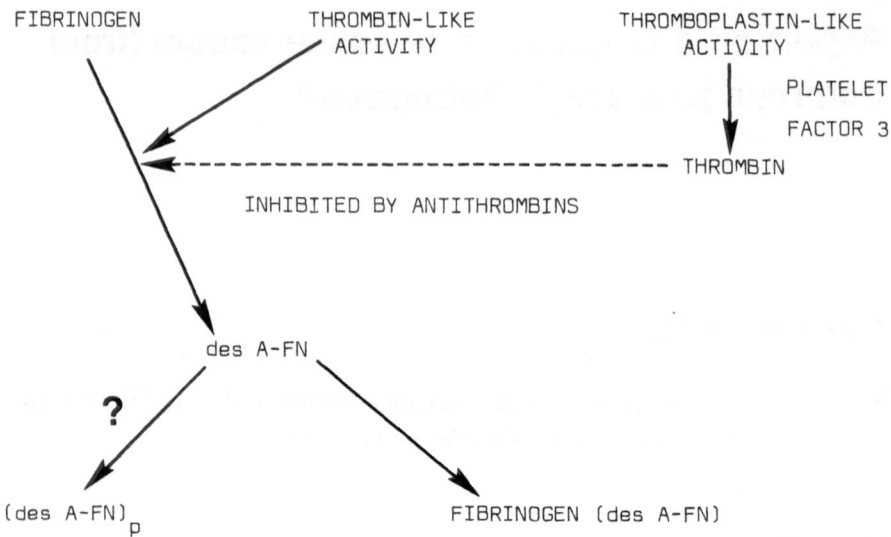

des A-FN: fibrin monomer which has been formed by the removal of fibrinopeptide A alone
from fibrinogen.

p: polymer.          *Fig. 1.* Proposed mode of action of Botropase®.

following the administration of high doses of the drug (approximately
1000 times the dose used in humans). To our knowledge no further
animal or human pharmacological data are available.

## Clinical efficacy in patients without a bleeding disorder

While a number of clinical studies have been conducted to test the
usefulness of Botropase® as a haemostatic agent during various types of
surgery, it was not possible to differentiate between its therapeutic and
prophylactic effectiveness. Clinical trials normally entailed the intravenous use of the drug prior to surgery while subsequent intramuscular
doses were given after surgery. Generally favourable results in connection with ENT surgery have been reported in uncontrolled trials
(Ottoboni and Ciurlo, 1957, *inter alia*). One double-blind trial (Nicoucar,
1975) has been recently reported in which 20 ENT patients were given
Botropase® prophylactically (i.v.) and therapeutically (i.m.) while 20
controls were given a placebo. This trial showed that significantly (p
<0.01) less haemorrhage was observed in the Botropase® treated group;
however the extent of blood loss was by a subjective visual observation

on a scale of 0-4. In a recent summary of the use of Botropase® as a haemostatic agent (Marti, 1975) the author suggests that the drug is useful in reducing blood loss postoperatively, particularly following ENT surgery. The efficacy of Botropase®, therapeutically used during ear microsurgery, has been recently reported using each patient as his own control before and after therapy and using an objective method of blood loss measurement (Delaruelle and Marquet, 1976). However, none of the studies reported would satisfy this symposium's definition of a double-blind controlled trial. Many investigations (not mentioned here) estimated the efficacy of the drug by a reduction of bleeding and whole blood clotting times, in conjunction with a subjective assessment of blood loss.

## Clinical efficacy in patients with a bleeding disorder

While an antihaemorrhagic effect of Botropase® has been claimed for a number of non-surgically induced cases of bleeding (haemophilia, internal and external haemorrhage from various organs) no data are available to our knowledge which would satisfy the conditions for a controlled double-blind trial. The efficacy of Botropase® has been claimed (Cazzola, 1957; Peck and Morris-Goldberger, 1933; Pescetto and Malagamba, 1959) in the treatment of menorrhagia and postpartum haemorrhage. However, these studies were highly subjective and ill-controlled.

## Side effects

No side effects attributable to the drug have been reported in the literature. However the report (Durante *et al.*, 1962) of high mortality among post-prostatectomy patients with cardiovascular complications who had received a similar coagulant drug (Reptilase®) must be noted.

## Recommended dose

1 ml dose i.v. followed by 1-2 ml daily. This dose regimen has been exceeded in many studies found in the literature with no reported cardiovascular side effects.

## Contraindications

Patients with venous or arterial thrombosis or other thrombophilic conditions; afibrinogenaemia and dysfibrinogenaemia.


## Conclusions

There is little doubt that Botropase® shortens the whole blood clotting time both *in vivo* and *in vitro*. However this drug cannot be recommended as a general haemostatic since it seems to depend for its effect on the induction of low grade disseminated intravascular coagulation (DIC) in the patient's plasma. The extent and complications of this drug-induced DIC would be impossible to predict and the possibility of a cardiovascular incident would always exist; this would be particularly so when the drug is used therapeutically. Furthermore, the use of this drug, whose effectiveness as a haemostatic has been mainly demonstrated only in the field of minor and micro-surgery, could possibly delay the use of more effective haemostatic regimens in cases of serious blood loss; such a delay could have serious consequences for the patient.

REFERENCES

BLOMBACK B., BLOMBACK M. and NILLSON L.M. (1957) Coagulation studies on Reptilase, an extract of the venom of Bothrops atrox. *Thrombos. Diathes. haemorrh. (Stuttg.)* 1, 76.

CAZZOLA D. (1957) Sull'impiego del veleno di Bothrops Jararaca come coagulante in ostetrica e ginecologia. *Ginec. Obstet. Méx.* 7, 12.

DELARUELLE J. and MARQUET J. (1976) Coagulant fractions of snake venom and the control of capillary bleeding during microsurgery of the ear. In vivo demonstration. *Arch. Otolaryng.* In press.

DE NICOLA P., GUCCIONE G., MANARA G. and CIPOLLI P.L. (1969) Manifestazioni emorragiche in pazienti con reperti normali dell emocoagulazione e dell'emostasi. *Minerva otorinolaring.* 17, 183.

DINELLI C.A., MONTANI E. and SALA E. (1959) Ricerche sperimentali in vitro sull'azione dell'emocoagulase del veleno di Bothrops Jararaca. *Haematologica* 355.

DURANTE L.J., MOUTSOS A., AMBROSE R.B., DUNCAN W.J., FLEMING W., ZINSSER H.H. and PHILLIPS L.L. (1962) Prostatectomy bleeding. *Ann. Surg.* 156, 781.

GIBELLI A. and GIAROLA P. (1973) Sulla standardizzazione delle frazioni coagulanti del veleno di Bothrops nella terapia antiemorragica. *Progr. Med. (Napoli)* 29, 805.

LAMPUGNANI A. and CULTRERA G. (1970) Effect of Bothrops Jararaca venom coagulant fraction on fibrinogen turnover. *Farmaco, Ed. sci.* 25, 985.

LEROY G. (1965) *Contribution à l'étude expérimentale des propriétés de la fraction coagulante P33 du venin de Bothrops jararaca.* Doctoral thesis, Paris.

MARTI Th. (1975) Zur praktischen Anwendung der blutgerinnenden Wirkung der Botropase. *Praxis* 64, 1323.

NICOUCAR G. (1975) L'utilisation prophylactique et therapeutique de la Botropase en chirurgie ORL. *Méd. et Hyg. (Genève)* 33, 772.

OTTOBONI A. and CIURLO E. (1957) Azione del veleno di Bothrops Jararaca come coagulante in O.R.L. *Minerva otorinolaring* 7, 4.

PECK S. and MORRIS-GOLDBERGER A. (1933) The treatment of uterine bleeding with snake venom. *Amer. J. Obstet. Gynec.* 25, 887.

PESCETTO G. and MALAGAMBA G. (1959) Sul meccanismo di azione del veleno di Bothrops Jararaca e sulle sue indicazioni in campo ginecologico. *Haematologica* 173.

STOCKER K. and STRAUB P.W. (1970) Rapid detection of fibrinopeptides by bidimentional paper electrophoresis. *Thrombos. Diathes. haemorrh. (Stuttg.)* 24, 248.

# Comments on Botropase®

by P. de Nicola, spokesman for Ravizza Co., Muggiò (Milan)

The active principle extracted from the venom of *Bothrops jararaca*, and contained in Botropase®, has been classified amongst those substances whose action is predominantly thrombin-like.

## The mechanism of action of Botropase®

The thrombin-like action of the active principle of *Bothrops jararaca* venom or Botropase® is characterized primarily by the fact that blood coagulation takes place even when all other clotting factors except fibrinogen are absent, in particular calcium, prothrombin and various other plasmatic and platelet factors.

In this way the action of Botropase® is similar to that of thrombin, which converts fibrinogen into fibrin without the intervention of any other factors. By injecting the animal with a solution of heparin, or a synthetic heparinoid substance, the blood becomes almost completely incoagulable. If, however, Botropase® is administered, either prior to or simultaneously with the other injection, coagulation of the blood takes place in normal or almost normal time (Rosenfeld *et al.*, 1962; de Nicola and Cappelletti, 1959).

There are, however, some significant differences between the mode of action of Botropase® and that of thrombin; the main ones are as follows:

(1) The action of thrombin can be inhibited by the antithrombin normally present in the blood, whereas the action of Botropase® continues, even when antithrombin III is present (de Nicola and Cappelletti, 1959);

(2) After either thrombin or Botropase® action, the terminal amino acids in the fibrin clots are tyrosine and glycine; however, whereas with thrombin the ratio is 1 : 2, with Botropase® it is 1 : 1 (Blombäck *et al.*, 1957);

(3) Unlike thrombin, Botropase® is not absorbed by the fibrin clots and is therefore not neutralized by this mechanism, as is thrombin.

The most important of these differences, from the practical point of view, is the fact that Botropase® remains in the blood stream even when antithrombin is present, and is not absorbed by fibrin clots; this enables the action of Botropase® to be much more prolonged than is possible with thrombin, which is immediately neutralised by fibrin clots.

Recent research has enabled the mode of action of *Bothrops jararaca* haemocoagulase to be more exactly defined. In the first place it has been noted (Dinelli *et al.*, 1959) that it is possible, by means of electrophoresis, to establish the direct action of Botropase® on fibrinogen.

As far as blood platelets are concerned, it has repeatedly been confirmed that when Botropase® comes into contact with them, it releases thromboplastic factors from them. This effect may be demonstrated by means of the thromboplastin generation test.

Finally, it is worth mentioning that the research carried out by Del Campo and Fazzi (1959) has shown that Botropase® is not antigenic and therefore specific antibodies are not formed after its injection.

## Tests to evaluate the toxicity of Botropase® in animals

Three different routes of administration are employed to evaluate the toxicity of Botropase® preparations (Ravizza Research Laboratories, unpublished data):
(1) 2ml (6.6 ml/kg) of undiluted solution are administered i.v. to pigeons weighing 300 g. The animals are kept under observation for 30 min.
(2) 5 ml (14.2-16.6 ml/kg) of undiluted solution are administered i.m. to guinea pigs weighing 300-350 g. The guinea pigs are kept under observation for 7 days.
(3) 5 ml of undiluted solution are administered subcutaneously to guinea pigs weighing 300-350 g. The guinea pigs are kept under observation for 7 days.

In none of the above-mentioned tests have the animals died or shown signs of general or local intolerance. For each route of administration 5 animals are used. Extensive studies on toxicity have been carried out by Leroy (1965).

## Standardization of Botropase®

For the exact characterization of Botropase® and its differentiation from other similar products, the most important feature is represented by its standardization in NIH thrombin units.

Comparative studies in this respect have been carried out by Gibelli and Giarola (1973). They have emphasized the possibility of using purified fibrinogen as a standard substrate for the titration of the thrombin-like action of Botropase®, and pointed out that by using plasma as a substrate, as suggested in other techniques, the results are not dependable enough, due to the presence in the plasma of several factors which cannot be exactly controlled and standardized. According to these authors, the presence of a thromboplastin-like activity in the haemocoagulse may interfere with the results when plasma is used as a substrate, especially if calcium is added to the coagulation mixture. These procedures do not, however, allow standardization of the coagulant activity in internationally accepted units. The thromboplastin-moiety is therefore not contained in the commercial preparations of Botropase®. If the predominant action of a coagulant drug is thrombin-like, as with Botropase®, the procedure of choice is to titrate it in NIH units.

The results obtained by Gibelli and Giarola (1973) clearly indicated that the thrombin-like activity of Botropase® is stronger than other products, if comparable commercial preparations are employed.

## The clinical use of Botropase®

The coagulant action of Botropase® was studied in animals, normal subjects and patients (haemophilic syndromes) using a number of blood coagulation tests: whole blood clotting time, recalcification time, thromboelastography, partial thromboplastin time etc. Under these conditions a reduction of the coagulation times in the tests concerned was observed.

It may be assumed, as a close approximation, that up to now several hundred thousand subjects have been treated with Botropase®, on the basis of the data of sales during the last years (IMFO 1972-1976).

The antihaemorrhagic effect of Botropase® has been studied in many clinical conditions: haemophilic syndromes and other primary and secondary haemorrhagic syndromes; postoperative haemorrhages and internal and external haemorrhages in various organs (haematomas, epistaxis, haemoptysis, gastrorrhagia, haematemesis, enterorrhagia, melaena, haematuria, meno and metrorrhagia, etc.).

Naturally in cases of life-threatening or severe haemorrhages, Botropase® should not be used as the prime and sole drug, but in association with transfusions and possibly with other haemostatic drugs. It is obvious that Botropase® is no substitute for blood transfusions when there is massive haemorrhage but it represents a valid and effective aid in the arrest of bleeding.

The antihaemorrhagic effect of Botropase® in ENT surgery was evaluated by Nicoucar (1975) in 20 patients, as compared with 20 patients given placebo. It was a double-blind, randomized trial.

From the statistical analysis of the results a significant difference was found between patients treated with Botropase® and untreated patients as far as total bleeding was concerned.

Particularly interesting are the investigations of Delaruelle and Marquet (1977) on the effect of Botropase® during microsurgery of the ear. According to the authors, the i.v. use of Botropase® proved to be highly effective in controlling the bleeding in 318 cases out of 398 (75%).

Botropase®, given intravenously (even in a single dose of 2-6 ampoules), was perfectly tolerated by all the patients without any side effects or allergic manifestations.


## Contraindications and untoward effects of Botropase®

The only situations in which Botropase® is contraindicated are thromboembolic diseases, thrombophilic states and disseminated intravascular coagulation syndromes.

In all other cases, the intravenous and intramuscular administration of Botropase®, even over a long period (weeks or months), is always perfectly well tolerated and has never been followed by intravascular coagulation or by the clinical manifestations of it.

Botropase® has a thrombin-like action, exclusively liberating fibrinopeptide A from the fibrinogen molecule and thus leading to circulating des-A-fibrin monomers. The presence of such circulating fibrin monomers (liberated physiologically in the first phase of action of thrombin) gives rise to positive paracoagulation tests and cryofibrinogenaemia. Even though, theoretically, such phenomena are signs of an incipient or latent intravascular coagulation, the usual therapeutic or prophylactic dose of Botropase® used is so small that it does not lead to clinical signs of disseminated intravascular coagulation (DIC). It is possible to obtain a manifest DIC by introducing 0.5-1 NIH units of Botropase®/kg in dogs, whereas the recommended dose in man is 1 vial (1 NIH unit) possibly followed by a second administration. Such a dose calculated for a man of 70 kg is about 0.015 NIH units of Botropase®/kg.

Moreover studies carried out with the venom from *Bothrops* in order to obtain intravascular defibrination in selected patients, using much higher doses than those usually recommended, were never followed by manifestations of DIC (Lampugnani and Cultrera, 1970). In the past twenty-five years, since the introduction of Botropase® for clinical use, about 60 million vials have been sold exclusively to hospitals, and up to now no complications or side-effects which might be due to DIC have been reported (data supplied by the manufacturer).

Taking into consideration the literature and the experience of physicians who have used Botropase®, it can be said with ease that even though in theory Botropase® acts by inducing a latent intravascular coagulation, in practice the use of Botropase® with the doses recommended by the manufacturer has never been followed by DIC.

The slow intravenous infusion of up to 6 vials of Botropase® (Lampugnani and Cultrera, 1970) was performed without any untoward effect. Also the prolonged intramuscular administration of Botropase® (up to three vials daily) was always well tolerated (Sannino *et al.* 1965). Of course, Botropase® has no effect in the presence of a severe fibrinogen deficiency (hypofibrinogenaemia, afibrinogenaemia).

REFERENCES

BLOMBACK B., BLOMBACK M, and NILSSON I.M. (1957) Coagulation studies on Reptilase, an extract of the venom from Bothrops Jararaca. *Thrombos. Diathes. haemorrh. (Stuttg.)* 1, 76.
DELARUELLE J. and MARQUET J. (1977) Coagulant fractions of snake venom and the control of capillary bleeding during microsurgery of the ear: in vivo demonstration. *Arch. Otolaryng.* 217.
DEL CAMPO A. and FAZZI P. L. (1959) Alcuni aspetti in immunologia e in batteriologia dell'emocoagulasi di Bothrops Jararaca. *Haematologica* 391.
DE NICOLA P. and CAPPELLETTI G. A. (1959) I processi di coagulazione e i veleni degli ofidi. Basi fisiopatologiche delle applicazioni diagnostiche e terapeutiche. *Haematologica* 17.

DINELLI C. A. et al. (1959) Ricerche sperimentali in vitro sull'azione dell'emocoagulase del veleno di Bothrops Jararaca. *Haematologica* 355.

GIBELLI A. and GIAROLA P. (1973) Sulla standardizzazione delle frazioni coagulanti del veleno di Bothrops nella terapia antiemorragica. *Progr. Med. (Napoli)* 29, 805.

IMFO (Il Mercato Farmaceutico Ospedaliero) Italia 1972 (p. 488), 1973 (p. 471), 1974 (p. 458), 1975 (p. 197), 1976 (p. 143).

LAMPUGNANI A. and CULTRERA G. (1970) Effect of Bothrops Jararaca venom coagulant fraction on fibrinogen turnover. *Farmaco, Ed. sci.* 25, 985.

LEROY G. (1965) *Contribution à l'étude expérimentale des propriétés de la fraction coagulante P33 du venin de Bothrops Jararaca.* Vigot Frères, Paris.

NICOUCAR G. (1975) L'utilisation prophylactique et thérapeutique de la Botropase en chirurgie O.R.L. *Méd. et Hyg. (Genève)* 33, 772.

ROSENFELD G., MARTINS L. F., GRECCHI R. and KELEN E. M. A. (1962) Neutralization of anticoagulant effect of heparin 'in vitro' and 'in vivo' by the coagulant fraction of snake venom (Bothrops Jararaca). In: *Proc. IX Internat. Congr. Haematology, Mexico.*

SANNINO M. et al. (1965). L'azione della frazione emocoagulante del veleno del Bothrops Jararaca sull'Herpes Zoster, sull'Herpes Simplex e sulla varicella. Prime esperienze clinico-terapeutische. *Minerva Med.* 56, 3681.

# Report on a preparation of snake venom (from Bothrops atrox): Reptilase®

## Chemical description

Reptilase® is a coagulant fraction of *B. atrox* venom. It contains two active coagulant principles, a thrombin-like calcium-independant activity and a thromboplastin-like activity. The thrombin-like enzyme is a glycopeptide of molecular weight 40,000 and, unlike thrombin which catalyses the hydrolytic removal of fibrinopeptide A and B from fibrinogen, it specifically removes only fibrinopeptide A from fibrinogen (Blombäck *et al.*, 1957; Stocker and Straub, 1970). The thromboplastin-like activity has a molecular weight of 66,000 and can generate thrombin in the presence of platelet factor 3.

## Mode of action

The thrombin-like enzyme in Reptilase® differs from thrombin as follows: (a) The known thrombin inhibitors, including heparin and hirudin, do not inhibit it (Blombäck *et al.*, 1957; Stocker and Straub, 1970), (b) the fibrin monomer formed contains fibrinopeptide B (Blombäck *et al.*, 1957) and (c) it activates factor XIII poorly. While thrombin is continuously inactivated in blood by circulating antithrombins, the thrombin-like activity in Reptilase®, which is not thus inhibited, can act even at a very low dose level. Thus low levels of Reptilase® can form a fibrin monomer (des-A type) which complexes with fibrinogen to yield a soluble fibrin monomer complex (SFMC) (Harder and Straub, 1972). This SFMC can readily be converted to a fibrin clot by thrombin. The role of SFMC in hypercoagulability has been questioned recently (Blattler *et al.*, 1974). These authors suggest that SFMC may not exist in blood at 37°C and are merely a laboratory artefact. A mechanism of action for the thromboplastin-like activity of Reptilase® could involve the generation of thrombin during platelet aggregation. Whereas a proven mode of action for Reptilase® *in vivo* remains unknown, the presence of SFMC and other indications of a hypercoagulable state (Harder *et al.*, 1972) following its administration to humans and animals would suggest that fibrin clot 'intermediates' have been formed which render blood more prone to coagulation. These mechanistic proposals are the same as those made for Botropase® (see Fig. 1, p. 90).

## Animal and human pharmacology

*Toxicity.* Mice, guinea-pigs and cats were given subcutaneous and intraperitoneal doses of Reptilase® which approximated to 100 times the recommended human dosage over periods of up to 30 days. The animals showed no symptoms of toxicity and microcospic examination of various tissues (brain, kidney, adrenals, spleen, heart, liver and lung) revealed no evidence of intravascular coagulation.

*Coagulation studies in animals.* A shortening of the whole blood clotting time in mice, rabbits, rats and monkeys was observed following injection of Reptilase®. The onset and the duration of this effect seemed to depend on the route of injection. The *in vivo* bleeding time of mice was reduced considerably by low doses of Reptilase®.

*Pharmacology.* Reptilase® has no effect either on the cardiovascular system or on the respiratory system of the rabbit. Neither was any direct effect on smooth muscle or neuromuscular conduction observed. High doses (100 times the recommended human dose) caused gross aberrations of the ECG trace of the cat which recoverd after 15 minutes.

*Antigenicity.* Results, using adult guinea-pigs sensitised by intradermal injections of Reptilase®, suggested that an anaphylactic reaction should not be expected with this drug.

## Clinical efficacy in patients without a bleeding disorder

Reptilase® has been used as a haemostatic in general, dental, and ENT surgery and in the field of obstetrics. Table 1 contains the salient features of the three double-blind controlled studies of the use of Reptilase® in association with surgically-induced blood loss. Many other clinical reports exist in the literature but could not be classified within the general meaning of double-blind. Indeed, the requirements for double-blind clinical trials by the organisers of the Leuven meeting were not fulfilled in any of these three studies in that there was no evidence presented that the control and test groups were equally prone to blood loss at the beginning of the study. To overcome this inter-individual variation and difficulty in studying adequately matched groups, large numbers would need to be included in a trial which would give statistically significant results.

One of the three double-blind studies (no. 3, Table 1) reported that Reptilase® had no significant effect on blood loss (during adenotonsil-lectomy) while the other two (nos. 1 and 2, Table 1) issued favourable reports. It must be conceded that the investigators in trial no. 3 gave more evidence of a randomised trial than those reporting favourably on Reptilase®. Despite the lack of double-blind studies, large numbers of observations on clotting and bleeding times suggest that Reptilase® renders blood more clottable *in vivo* and *in vitro*. Whether this in turn affects the blood loss in all cases of haemorrhage is not wholly evident. Only one instance of Reptilase® being of possible therapeutic value during a life-threatening haemorrhage has come to our attention (Blombäck, unpublished data, 1972). The cumulative, rather subjective, experience with Reptilase® over the last 20 years has suggested (Stacher and Bohnel, 1959; Durante *et al.* 1962; Sugano and Muruyama, 1964, *inter alia*) that the drug has a haemostatic effect during the bleeding particularly associated with ENT surgery. However, the intravenous use of Reptilase® to combat such minor bleeding could not be recommended in the light of the possible hazards to the patient from some form of intravascular coagulation associated with the proven induction of a hypercoagulable state in the circulating plasma. While no great general incidence of cardiovascular complications associated with the use of

Table 1. Double-blind controlled clinical studies using Reptilase® as a haemostatic agent

| No. | Author | Application in | No. of patients | | Haemostatic effect | Objective measure of blood loss |
|-----|--------|----------------|------|------|------|------|
| | | | Treated | Control | | |
| 1 | Hirasugi *et al.* 1973 | Otorhinolaryngology | 29 | 27 | Yes | Yes |
| 2 | Burke *et al.* 1960 | Prostatectomy | 48 | 50 | Yes | Yes |
| 3 | Verstraete *et al.* 1977 | Adenotonsillectomy | 64 | 65 | No | Yes |

Reptilase® is evident from the literature, the study of Durante *et al.* (1962) concluded that clotting agents used as haemostatics during prostatectomy increase the mortality rate among patients with postoperative cardiovascular complications. The same authors observed that Reptilase® reduced bleeding significantly (at 0.05 level) only after transurethral resection.

## Clinical efficacy in patients with a bleeding disorder

The most common type of bleeding diathesis encountered is that associated with heavy menstrual bleeding (menorrhagia). Picha *et al.* (1957) have reported that H-6102®[1] did not appear to be effective in the treatment of menorrhagia and metrorrhagia while Laralde and Labat (1965) reported that the drug is effective in reducing menstrual bleeding. A number of cases have been reported (Ohlenschlager and Schwalbe, 1966) in which various haemorrhagic diatheses (due to antibody formation, lymphatic and myeloid leukaemia) have been favourably treated with Reptilase®. None of these was a controlled double-blind study.

It has been suggested that Reptilase® might be of use in the treatment of haemophilic patients. Harder *et al.* (1972) compared various clotting parameters in five haemophiliacs, treated with Reptilase®, using ten normal controls, five of whom were given a placebo. Apart from the observation that Reptilase® caused a type of low grade intravascular coagulation, Reptilase® induced raised factor VIII levels while no such enhancement was noted with the haemophiliac group. All the Reptilase®-treated controls and haemophiliacs showed reduced clotting times in conjuction with positive paracoagulation tests which were followed by a lowering of the fibrinogen levels and an elevation of the fibrinogen degradation products (FDP) level. The drastic reduction in the prothrombin in some haemophiliacs could suggest that some fibrin intermediates may have an activating effect on other components in the clotting system (Gaffney and Brasher 1974). No enhancement of fibrinolytic activity was noticed in either group despite the lowered fibrinogen and elevated FDP levels. It was concluded that Reptilase® acted directly on fibrinogen in shortening the plasma clotting time but no opinion was offered on the influence of the des-A-fibrin monomers on the

1. H-6102®: a preparation of venoms from *Bothrops jararaca* and *Lachesis atrox*.

haemostatic effectiveness attributed to Reptilase®. These authors (Harder *et al.*, 1972) suggested a trial of Reptilase® to evaluate its effectiveness in combatting the haemorrhagic episodes of haemophiliacs. A very limited trial (Verstraete, 1973, unpublished data) using five haemophiliacs and one control suggested that Reptilase® did not affect the clotting tests.

This brief résumé of Reptilase® as a therapy in non-surgically induced blood loss does not allow any clear conclusion on its effectiveness as a haemostatic agent.

## Side effects

No side effects directly attributable to this drug have been cited in the literature. However, there is an increased mortality rate among patients (mostly aged patients undergoing prostatectomy) with postoperative cardiovascular complications who had been given the drug compared to those with similar postoperative complications who had not been given the drug (Durante *et al.*, 1962).

## Recommended dose

Normally 1 ampoule (1 ml), usually intravenously, followed by 1-2 ampoules daily given intramuscularly. (Variation according to use i.e. whether as a prophylactic before surgery or during emergency haemorrhage).

## Contraindications

Patients with venous or arterial thrombosis or other thrombophilic conditions; afibrinogenaemia and dysfibrinogenaemia.

## Conclusions

There is little doubt that Reptilase® shortens the whole blood clotting time both *in vivo* and *in vitro* and three out of four double-blind studies suggested that it was effective as a haemostatic. However this drug cannot be recommended as a general haemostatic since it seems to depend for its effect on the induction of low grade disseminated intravascular coagulation (DIC) in the patient's plasma. The extent and complications of this drug induced DIC would be impossible to predict and the possibility of a cardiovascular incident would always exist; this would be particularly so when the drug is used therapeutically. Furthermore, the use of this drug, whose effectiveness as a haemostatic has been mainly demonstrated in the field of minor and microsurgery, could possibly delay the use of more effective haemostatic regimens in cases of serious blood loss; such a delay could have serious consequences for the patient.

## REFERENCES

BLATTLER W., STRAUB P.W. and PAYER A. (1974) Effect of in vivo produced fibrinogen-fibrin intermediates on viscosity of human blood. *Thrombos. Res.* 4, 787.

BLOMBACK B., BLOMBACK M. and NILSSON I.M. (1957) Coagulation studies on 'Reptilase' an extract of the venom from Bothrops jararaca. *Thrombos. Diathes. haemorrh. (Stuttg.)* 1, 76.

BURKE D.E., POGRUND R.S. and CLARK W.G. (1960) Haemostatic agents in control of bleeding. *Clin. Res.* 8, 127 (Abstr.)

DURANTE L.J., MOUTSOS A., AMBROSE R.B., DUNCAN W.J., FLEMING W., ZINSSER H.H. and PHILLIPS L.L. (1962) Prostatectomy bleeding. *Ann. Surg.* 156, 781.

GAFFNEY P.J. and BRASHER M. (1974) Mode of action of ancrod as a defibrinating agent. *Nature (Lond.)* 251, 53.

HARDER A.J. and STRAUB P.W. (1972) In vitro and in vivo induction of cryofibrinogen and 'paracoagulation' by Reptilase. *Thrombos. Diathes. haemorrh. (Stuttg.)* 27, 337.

HARDER A.J., STADELMANN H. and STRAUB P.W. (1972) Reptilase-induced shortening of coagulation times in normal and hemophilic individuals. *Thrombos. Diathes. haemorrh.* (Stuttg.) 27, 349.

HIRASUGI Y., OHYAMA S., INOUE Y. and YASUNO T. (1973) Clinical experience with Reptilase-S injection. *Jap. J. Clin. Report* 7, 157.

LARRALDE CH. and LABAT M. (1965) Etude clinique d'un nouvel hémostatique en gynécologie chirurgicale et médicale. *J. méd. Bordeaux* 1.

OHLENSCHLAGER G. and SCHWALBE J. (1966) Klinische Erfahrungen mit Reptilase bei hämorrhagischen Diathesen und post-operativen Blutungen. *Med. Mschr.* 20, 179.

PICHA E.A., ROCHENSCHAUB A. and WEGHAUPT K. (1957) Beitrag zur hämostatischen Behandlung in der operativen und honservativen gynakologie. *Wien. med. Wschr.* 107, 74.

STACHER A. and BOHNEL J. (1959) Experimentelle und klinische Untersuchungen zur hämostatischen Wirkung von Schlangengiften. *Wien. klin. Wschr.* 19, 333.

STOCKER K. and STRAUB P.W. (1970) Rapid detection of fibrinopeptides by bidimensional paper electrophoresis. *Thrombos. Diathes. haemorrh. (Stuttg.)* 24, 248.

SUGANO T. and MARUYAMA R. (1964) Experience of the use of Reptilase in the field of otorhinolaryngology. *Otorhinolaryngology (Tokyo)*, 36, 363.

VERSTRAETE M., TYBERGHEIN J., DE GREEF Y., DAEMS L. and VAN HOOF A. (1977) Double-blind trials with ethamsylate, Batroxobin or tranexamic acid on blood loss after adenotonsillectomy. *Acta clin. Belg.* 32, 136.

# Comments by the manufacturer of Reptilase®

**by K. Stocker, Pentapharm Ltd., CH-4002 Basle**

Manipulation of plasma fibrinogen by parenteral administration of thrombin[1] or thrombin-like snake-venom enzymes[2], in low doses, is being used to favour haemostasis and, in high doses[3], to cause blood incoagulability by complete fibrinogen depletion.

During the past 20 years nearly 100 million ampoules of Reptilase® have been given by thousands of qualified physicians to millions of patients; moreover thousands of patients have been defibrinogenated with thrombin-like snake-venom enzymes.

Side-effects have rarely been attributed to Reptilase®; only 3 out of 41 original publications contain these reports: Durante *et al.* (1962) registered the death of 2 out of 5 risk-patients who underwent prostatectomy under Reptilase® medication, whereas only 12 out of 53 died in the control group. Hafter and Graeff (1975) attributed aggravation of diffuse intravascular coagulation during the course of dead fetus syndrome to Reptilase® and Soria *et al.* (1977) observed symptoms of allergic shock in one patient following prolonged Reptilase® treatment.

Defibrinogenation which is preceeded by the complete conversion of plasma-fibrinogen into des-A-type fibrin monomer, has proved to be a safe procedure regardless of whether fibrin related material is present during the hours following intravenous application or during several days following subcutaneous injection of thrombin-like snake-venom enzymes.

The thrombin-like action of Reptilase® is strictly limited to the Aα chain of fibrinogen (Aronson, 1976). Unlike thrombin, Reptilase® does not split off peptide B, does not activate platelets, and circulating Reptilase® does not consume antithrombin III. Thus, the narrow proteolytic action of Reptilase® on the Aα-chain differs definitely from the cascade of reactions and from the feed-back phenomena which

1. Thrombase®
2. Botropase®, Reptilase®
3. Arwin®, Defibrase®

characterize the fatal role of thrombin in diffuse intravascular coagulation. The *in vivo* action of Reptilase® may therefore be characterized as a definite and limited step towards coagulation rather than as a low-grade intravascular coagulation.

The distinct differences between the restricted action of Reptilase® and the role of thrombin in intravascular coagulation are reflected in the high degree of safety in its application which in consequence has allowed a broad clinical experience over decades. This fact ought to be considered in conjuction with the experts' recommendations.

REFERENCES

ARONSON D.L. (1976) Comparison of the actions of thrombin and the thrombin-like venom enzymes Ancrod and Batroxobin. *Thrombos. Haemostas. (Stuttg.)* 36, 9.

DURANTE J., MOURSOS A., AMBROSE R.B., DUNCAN Y., FLEMING W. and PHILLIPS L. (1962) Postprostatectomy bleeding: analysis and consequences of control by clotting agents and hypothermia. *Ann. Surg.* 156, 781.

HAFTER R. and GRAEFF H. (1975) Molecular aspects of defibrination in a Reptilase-treated case of dead fetus syndrome. *Thrombos. Res.* 7, 391.

SORIA J., SORIA C., VINAZZER H. and STOCKER K. (1977) A tanned red cell haemagglutination immuno-assay for the estimation of antibodies directed against defibrase. *Thrombos. Res.* 10, 623.

# Report on aprotinin[1]: Trasylol®

Trasylol® is today a therapeutic challenge not only in the field of haematology but in other clinical fields. While its structure, pharmacology and activity has been studied exhaustively in the past decade in a wide variety of experimental situations, a great deal of data relates to experimental studies in animals and its use in the treatment of disease in man is still ill defined.

## Chemical definition

Isolated from bovine lung, this serine protease inhibitor has a defined molecular weight of 6,512. It is identical to the basic pancreatic trypsin inhibitor described by Kunitz in 1936. It is made up of 16 different amino acids making up a chain of 58 amino acids, the active centre being in the lysine-15 site. (Werle, 1968 and 1971).

The inhibitory effect of Trasylol® on serine proteases (trypsin, plasmin, kallikrein and chymotrypsin) is due to an enzyme-substrate complex employing the active serine site of the enzyme in the normal way (Lazdunski et al., 1974). The combination with these proteases, shows, however, certain differences of the dissociation contants, the binding with trypsin being the most stable $(6 \times 10^{-14})$. The link with plasmin and kallikrein is similar but less stable and therefore possibly reversible, dissociation constants being $2.3 \times 10^{-10}$ and $1 \times 10^{-7}$ respectively. The activity of Trasylol® is expressed as kallikrein inhibitor units (KIU), 1 unit being that which inhibits 2 kallikrein units by 50%;

Following the injection of Trasylol® in man there is an initial rapid clearance from the circulation followed by a steady exponential loss. This biphasic curve represents equilibration with the extravascular compartment and rapid renal uptake in the first 60 minutes (Just, 1975; Just et al., 1975). The true elimination of the drug can be deduced from the second slower part of the curve. From this data an overall blood half-life of 37-50 minutes can be deduced with a half-life of elimination of 150 minutes (Beller et al., 1966).

Trasylol® is not excreted unchanged in the urine and it is metabolised by the kidney, split products being released into the blood or urine.

1. Other preparations of aprotinin: Antagosan®, Iniprol®, Zymofren®.

## Mode of action

The inhibitory action of Trasylol® on various enzyme systems is reflected in its diverse activity in several biological systems.

*Fibrinolytic system.* Trasylol® appears to act as a specific inhibitor of active plasmin (McNicol *et al.*, 1969) but also on the conversion of plasminogen by activator (Ambrus *et al.*, 1968; Beck *et al.*, 1963).

While the synthetic inhibitors have similar activities, their mode of action is different.

*Coagulation sequence.* Trasylol® has an anticoagulant effect, its action being specifically directed against the contact sequence. (Blombäck *et al.*, 1967; Prentice *et al.*, 1970).

This sequence depends on the activation of factor XII (Hageman factor) which together with two other co-factors in turn activates factor XI. These co-factors have been recognised to be prekallikrein or kallikreininogen (Fletcher factor) and kininogen (Fitzgerald factor). When kallikrein is produced it in turn activates kininogen to kinins – both reactions being neutralised by Trasylol® and both playing a part in the fibrinolytic activator pathway as well as in the contact sequence (Back, 1966; Cochrane *et al.*, Colman, 1974; Wuepper, 1973; Waldmann *et al.*, 1975).

While this inhibitory effect of Trasylol® has a considerable effect *in vitro* it is doubtful whether there is any significant biological effect *in vivo* (Laake *et al.*, 1974).

Other effects on the coagulation sequence have been claimed:

(1) Prevention of the post-operation decrease of antihrombin III (Olsson and Nordstrom, 1964).

(2) Potentiation of the effect of thrombin on fibrinogen (Nordstrom *et al.*, 1968; Nordstrom and Zetterquist, 1968).

(3) In an experimental situation in rats it appears to reduce the amount of fibrin deposited in the lungs when an intravenous injection of thromboplastin is given. Trasylol® did not decrease the amount of lung fibrin produced by thrombin (Diffang and Saldeen, 1974).

*Kinin system.* As well as the anticoagulant effect described above, Trasylol has been shown to have an effect on the following:

(1) Experimental local Schwartzman reaction

(2) Oedema

(3) Pain

(4) Cell membrane integrity

(5) Infection and consequent 'shock' (endotoxin) as well as 'shock' produced by burns and scalding (Hey and Langer, 1971).

The beneficial effect induced by Trasylol® in these situations almost certainly relates to the inhibition of kinin formation and thus their effect on tissues and vessels.

*Trypsin.* The very strong avidity of Trasylol® for trypsin has little physiological significance but has been used to treat the effects of trypsin release from the pancreas in acute pancreatitis (see below).

## Clinical use of Trasylol®

*Patients with abnormal bleeding.* In this group it is the antifibrinolytic (antiplasmin) effect that is being utilised. Trasylol® has been recommended for use mainly in the acute acquired defects of the coagulation mechanism arising secondary to a variety of clinical situations.

*Obstetrics.* Any diffuse intravascular coagulation (DIC) episode in pregnancy e.g. abruptio placentae, amniotic fluid embolism and septic abortion.

When bleeding develops in these situations 'excessive fibrinolysis' is thought to be a factor – the latter situation being considered to exist if therapy with plasma or fibrinogen fails to improve the fibrinogen level or when the euglobulin lysis time continues to be less than 30 minutes.

Secondary effects of Trasylol® in the treatment of obstetric haemorrhage could be (a) to enhance the contraction of uterine muscle and (b) to inhibit vasodilation in uterine vessels – both effects being the result of inhibiting excess kinin production (Amris and Kjeldsen, 1966; Amris and Hilden, 1967; Beller and Epstein, 1968; Sher, 1974, 1975).

While the anticoagulant property of Trasylol® in these situations does not have any proven effect on the evidence available to date, there is equally no evidence that Trasylol® has any potentiating and perhaps deleterious effect on the induced coagulation sequence in these syndromes.

Most reports in the literature describe what can only be called anecdotal case histories, where the use of Trasylol® has produced an apparent dramatic effect in the individual. However, these are not balanced by controls and clinical trials to substantiate these claims.

*DIC in other clinical syndromes.* The comments made above apply to the majority of episodes of DIC secondary to other disease.

Two possible exceptions are:
(1) DIC as a consequence of the endotoxaemia associated with a Gram-negative septicaemia.
(2) purpura gangrenosa.

Based on experimental data, Trasylol® may ameliorate the endotoxin shock syndrome and gross pain and oedema of purpura gangrenosa.

In both instances the use of this drug would be secondary to the use of antibiotics and/or anticoagulants. Again no acceptable trials have been carried out.

*Post-surgical bleeding.* In one large randomised trial (Matis, 1967) Trasylol® was tested in a four group trial (1,000 patients/group): (a) Control. (b) Marcoumar®. (c) Marcoumar®/Trasylol®. (d) Trasylol®. Trasylol® was given in a dose of 1.3 million KIU over 72 hours postoperatively.

Randomised entry to the groups was achieved by using odd and even dates of birth. The groups were said to evenly match in terms of age and types of surgery. When both the Trasylol® and Marcoumar®/Trasylol® group were compared with the other two groups there appeared to be a marginal but significant reduction in the incidence of wound haematoma and wound infection in the former groups and an increased rate of healing. Mortality attributed to pulmonary embolism was also reduced by 50% in groups where Trasylol® was used. Trasylol® was ineffective in stopping bleeding post-prostatectomy where excess local fibrinolysis can be demonstrated (Smutzler and Furstenberg, 1966).

## Other clinical uses of Trasylol®

*Acute pancreatitis* (Trapnell *et al.*, 1974). Recent trials have demonstrated the beneficial effects of Trasylol® in acute pancreatitis provided it is given early in the clinical course and in sufficient dosage. Further randomised double-blind trials are underway.

*Prevention of post-operative deep vein thrombosis.* Trasylol® has been shown to improve the speed of venous blood flow in the leg in the post-operative period by promoting venous constriction and arterial dilatation and thus enhancing venous blood flow (Rieckert *et al.*, 1969). The enhancement of antithrombin III levels mentioned above may also be beneficial in this situation.

Again these observations have not been put to adequate clinical test.

*Allergic phenomenon.* Trasylol® inhibits the kinin release consequent upon antigen-antibody reactions (anaphylactoid shock; delayed hypersensitivity reaction) and by so doing ameliorates the clinical manifestations of these reactions (Back *et al.*, 1965; Kalaydjuev *et al.*, 1969). Whether this inhibitor produces this effect by masking certain facets of these reactions e.g. bronchospasm or urticarial weal, or by a direct effect on the antigen-antibody trigger, is not clear.

*Fat embolism.* There is no direct conclusive evidence that Trasylol® has any beneficial effect in this syndrome (Gurd, 1971).

*Shock lung* (adult respiratory distress syndrome, DIC lung). Matis and Haberland (1973) suggest that heparin or induced lytic therapy in this syndrome may promote vascular permeability and thus worsen the clinical state. Therefore, Trasylol® used in addition would be expected to neutralise the permeability.

McMichan (1976) has described a well designed double-blind trial into the uses of aprotinin (Trasylol®) in post-trauma syndrome. 35 patients were given Trasylol® and 35 patients received an unspecified placebo. The trial period was 96 hours, starting as soon after admission as possible. Both groups were matched for age, sex and degree of injury.

The author claims that the incidence of respiratory insufficiency post-trauma was reduced by Trasylol® and that when stored blood was given there was a direct relationship with the volume of stored blood and the severity of pulmonary insufficiency. Again Trasylol® produced a significant reduction of this complication in patients receiving more than one litre of stored blood.

There was no difference in the amount of blood transfused between the two groups or in the amount of fat detected in the blood.

The Trasylol® group showed a higher platelet count and decreased pulmonary platelet trapping and lower blood triglyceride and lactate levels. All these latter factors are probably related to the mechanism or mechanisms, as yet unknown, that lead to improvement of pulmonary function in these patients. It is intriguing to suggest they could be related to the decrease of vascular permeability as suggested by Matis and Haberland.

McMichan (1976) concludes by recommending the prophylactic use of Trasylol® in the management of post-traumatic syndrome.

*Extracorporeal circulation in open heart surgery.* While studies by Mammen (1974) and Tsuji *et al.* (1974) show that Trasylol® could be shown to reduce fibrinolytic activity during by-pass, the drug had little effect on the levels of coagulation factors or the incidence of post-operative bleeding. While reduction of lytic activity might appear to be desirable there is no evidence whatever that this is so.

Nagaoka and Latori, 1975, propose a different reason to use Trasylol® in this situation. They suggest that Trasylol® will improve perfusion by maintaining peripheral vascular resistance and reducing permeability by reducing kininogen activation.

Normally active kinins are destroyed by passage through the lung but in a by-pass situation, this mechanism is neutralized and significant and perhaps deleterious kinin levels are maintained.

Again no satisfactory trials have been carried out but many problems of prolonged extracorporeal by-pass and perfusion have yet to be solved and further studies are certainly indicated.

*Myocardial infarction.* In recent experimental studies, Trasylol® was shown to reduce the degree of tissue damage consequent on the induction in animals of experimental coronary thrombosis (Lefer and Spath, 1975; Wilkens *et al.*, 1975). The results suggested that Trasylol®, by inhibiting kinin formation, indirectly protects the cell from anoxic damage and maintains cell wall integrity by neutralizing the kinin release in, or from, damaged tissue. While no claim has been made for the use of Trasylol® in the treatment of myocardial infarction in man, these observations are so intriguing as to suggest that further research into the effect of this enzyme inhibitor on cell injury might be worthwhile. Similar results have been reported by Cara *et al.* (1971) following anaesthesia.

## Side effects

Trasylol® has remarkably few recorded side effects – three cardiac arrests were recorded in some 2,000 patients receiving i.v. Trasylol® following surgery (Matis, 1967) – this incidence is not significant in this number of surgical patients.

Occasional hypersensitivity rashes have occurred, and recently severe anaphylaxis has been reported in one patient where the reaction was associated with the use of Trasylol® on two occasions (Proud and Chamberlain, 1976). These authors stress the need for skin testing. These allergic manifestations are odd in that Trasylol® has been reported to be of value in the treatment of such reactions.

There is no evidence that the inhibitory effect on plasmin has led to excess fibrin formation which has been deleterious.

## Conclusions

No definite evidence exists to date to prove that Trasylol® can, by inhibiting lysis, decrease blood loss. While beneficial results have been reported in individual patients, no acceptable trials are yet available in this context. Adequate controlled and randomized double-blind trials are difficult to design and manage in many of the clinical situations under discussion. Yet until they are done no definite guide-lines can be given for the use of this drug or the amount of it to be given in the management of excessive blood loss.

The exact role of serine protease enzyme inhibitors is difficult to define in health or disease. Whether these enzymes are beneficial and protective in one situation and deleterious in another must await the results of further study.

Two acceptable trials have been carried out which show a definite benefit following the use of Trasylol® in therapy:
(1) acute pancreatitis
(2) post-traumatic syndrome with reference to respiratory insufficiency.

The growing interest in the observations that Trasylol® apparently protects cells from anoxic damage is exciting and it is in this direction that further research should be directed.

In 1969 McNicol et al. stated that 'Trasylol® is an immensely interesting potent preparation with multiple effects on biological systems and may have a role in haematology. A plea must be made that this drug is still in the clinical investigation field and as many observations as possible should be made to determine its application to therapy. To this end well designed clinical trials are urgently needed'.

With the exceptions mentioned above this statement still holds true to date.

## REFERENCES

AMBRUS C.M., AMBRUS J.L., LASSMAN H.B. and MINK I.B. (1968) Studies on the mechanism of action of inhibitors of the fibrinolysin system. *Ann. N.Y. Acad. Sci.* 146, 430.

AMRIS C.J. and KJELDSEN J. (1966) Haemorrhagic diathesis due to abruptio placentae treated with Trasylol. *Acta obstet. gynec. scand.* 45, 180.

AMRIS C.J. and HILDEN M. (1967) Inhibition of thromboplastic activity by Trasylol. *Scand. J. Haemat.* 4, 3.

BACK N. (1966) Fibrinolysin system and vasoactive kinins. *Fed. Proc.* 25, 77.

BACK N., WILKENS H., MUNSON A.E. and STEGER R. (1965) Trasylol in experimental shock states. In: *Neue Aspekte der Trasylol Therapie. Bericht über ein internationales Symposion in Grosse Ledder.* (Gross R., and Kroneberg G., eds.) pp. 170-175, F.K. Schattauer Verlag, Stuttgart.

BECK E., SMUTZLER R. and DUCKERT F. (1963) Inhibition of fibrinolysis and fibrinogenolysis in man; EACA and kallikrein inhibitor. *Thrombos. Diathes. haemorrh. (Stuttg.)* 10, 106.

BELLER F.K., EPSTEIN M.D. and KALLER H. (1966) Distribution, half life time and placental transfer of the protease inhibitor Trasylol. *Thrombos. Diathes. haemorrh. (Stuttg.)* 16, 3. 3.

BELLER F.K. and EPSTEIN M.D. (1968) Indications and rationale for the use of proteinase inhibitors in obstetrics. *Ann. N.Y. Acad. Sci.* 146, 673.

BLOMBACK B., BLOMBACK M. and OLSSON P. (1967) Action of a proteolytic enzymatic inhibitor on blood coagulation in vitro. *Thrombos. Diathes. haemorrh. (Stuttg.)* 18, 2.

CARA M., POISVERT M., MIGNE J., DERAS C., LOUVILLE Y., HERMAN B., ROUSSEL J. and VEDRINE M.Y. (1971) Système des kinines, histamine, isoenzymes de la laetico – dehydrogenase en anesthésie – réanimation. In: *Proc. 21st Congr. Franç. Anesth. Reanon, Marseille*, p. 118.

COCHRANE C.G., REVAK S.D. and WUEPPER K.D. (1973) Hageman factor in solid and fluid phases – a critical role of kallikrein. *J. exp. Med.* 138, 1564.

COLMAN R.W. (1974) Formation of human plasma kinin. *New Engl. J. Med.* 291, 509.

DIFFANG C. and SALDEEN T. (1974) Effect of Trasylol on fibrin deposition and elimination in the lungs of rats with intravascular coagulation induced by thrombin or thromboplastin. *Thromb. Res.* 5, 263.

GURD A.R. (1971) Treatment of fat embolism. In: *New Aspects of Trasylol Therapy. Protease Inhibition in Shock Therapy. Report on an International Symposium.* (Brendel W. and Haberland G.L., eds.) pp. 137-140, F.K. Schattauer Verlag, Stuttgart.

HEY D. and LANGER P. (1971) Heparin, plasmin, EACA and Trasylol in scalding shock. In: *New Aspects of Trasylol Therapy. Protease Inhibition in Shock Therapy. Report on an International Symposium.* (Brendel W. and Haberland G.L., eds.) pp. 271-284, F.K. Schattauer Verlag, Stuttgart.

JUST M. (1975) In vivo inter-reaction of the Kunitz protease inhibitor and of insulin with subcellular structures from rat renal cortex. *Naunyn Schmiedeberg's Arch. Pharmak. exp. Path.* 289, 85.

JUST M., ROCKEL A., STANJEK A. and BODE F. (1975) Is there any tubular reabsorption of filtered proteins in rat kidney? *Naunyn-Schmiedeberg's Arch. Pharmak. exp. Path.* 289, 229.

KALAYDJUEV V., PETRUNOV B. and KOSTURKOV G. (1969) The influence of protease inhibitors on the production of antibodies and allergic reactions in test animals. In: *Proteases and Antiproteases in Cardioangiology.* p. 207, F.K. Schattauer Verlag, Stuttgart.

LAAKE K. and VENNEROD A.M. (1974) Factor XII-induced fibrinolysis: studies on the separation of pre-kallikrein, plasminogen pro-activator and factor XI in human plasma. *Thrombos. Res.* 4, 285.

LAZDUNSKI M., VINCENT J.P., SCHWEITZ H., PERON-RENNER M. and PUDLES J. (1974) Mechanism of association of trypsin (or chymotrypsin) with the pancreatic trypsin inhibitors (Kunitz and Kazal). Kinetics and thermodynamics of the interaction. In: *Proteinase Inhibitors.* (Fritz, H., Tschesche H., Greene L.J. and Truscheit E., eds.) pp. 420-431, Springer Verlag, Berlin.

LEFER A.M. and SPATH J.A. (1975) Protective effect of protease inhibition in myocardial ischaemia. In: *New Aspects of Trasylol Therapy. Experimental Myocardial Infarction. Report on an International Symposium.* (Cantin M., Haberland G.L., Schnells, G. and Selye H., eds.) pp. 311-328, F.K. Schattauer Verlag, Stuttgart.

McMICHAN J.C. (1976) *Post traumatic syndrome.* D. Phil. Thesis, Monash University, Melbourne.

McNICOL G.P., PRENTICE C.R.M. and DOUGLAS A.S. (1969) Trasylol and failure of haemostasis. In: *Proteases and Antiproteases in Cardiology.* pp. 89, F.K. Schattauer Verlag, Stuttgart.

MAMMEN E.F. (1974) Natural proteinase inhibitors in extracorporeal circulation. *Ann. N. Y. Acad. Sci.* 146, 754.

MATIS P. (1967) Effect of Trasylol on blood clotting and wound healing. In: *New Aspects of Trasylol Therapy. Reports on Symposia in Bad Godesberg and in Munich.* (Marx R., Imdahl H. and Haberland G.L., eds.) pp. 21-42, F.K. Schattauer Verlag, Stuttgart.

MATIS P. and HABERLAND G.L. (1973) The lung in shock. In: *New Aspects of Trasylol Therapy. The Lung in Shock. Report on an International Symposium.* (Haberland G.L. and Lewis D.H., eds.) pp. 259-269, F.K. Schattauer Verlag, Stuttgart.

NAGAOKA H. and LATORI M. (1975) Inhibition of kinin formation by a kallikrein inhibitor during extra corporeal circulation in open heart surgery. *Circ.* 52, 325.

NORDSTROM S., BLOMBACK B., BLOMBACK M., OLSSON P. and ZETTERQUIST E. (1968) Experimental investigation of the anti-thromboplastic and anti-fibrinolytic activity of Trasylol. *Ann. N.Y. Acad. Sci.* 146, 701.

NORDSTROM S. and ZETTERQUIST E. (1968) Effect of thrombin infusions on $^{131}$I-labelled fibrinogen in dogs. *Acta physiol. Scand.* 72, 75.

OLSSON P. and NORDSTROM S. (1964) The significance of post op variations in antithrombins. *Thorax Chirurgie und. Vaskulare Chirurgie* 12, 176.

PRENTICE C.R.M., McNICOL G.P. and DOUGLAS A.S. (1970) Studies on the anticoagulant action of aprotinin (Trasylol). *Thrombos. Diathes. haemorrh.* (Stuttg.) 24, 265.

PROUD G. and CHAMBERLAIN J. (1976) Anaphylactic reaction to aprotinin. *Lancet* ii, 48.

RIECKERT H., PAUSCHINGER P. and MATIS P. (1969) Effects of proteinase inhibitor on the periheral circulation. In: *Proteases and Antiproteases in Cardiology.* p. 175. F.K. Schattauer Verlag, Stuttgart.

SHER G. (1974) Trasylol in cases of accidental haemorrhage with coagulation disorder and associated uterine inertia. *S. Afr. med. J.* 48, 1452.

SHER G. (1975) The diagnosis and management of accidental haemorrhage with associated coagulopathy. *S. Afr. med. J.* 49, 1383.

SMUTZLER R. and FURSTENBERG H. (1966) Fibrinolysis and blood loss after surgery of the prostate and its response to anti-fibrinolysis. *Dtsch. med. Wschr.* 18, 297.

TRAPNELL J.E., RIGBY C.C. and TALBOT C.H. (1974) A controlled trial of Trasylol in the treatment of acute pancreatitis. *Brit. J. Surg.* 61, 177.

TSUJI H.K., REDINGTON J.V., KAY J.H. and GROESSWALD R.K. (1974) The study of fibrinolytic and coagulation factors during open heart surgery. *Ann. N.Y. Acad. Sci.* 146, 763.

WALDMANN R., ABRAHAM J.P., REBUCK J.W., CALDWELL J., SAITO H. and RATNOFF O.D. (1975) Fitzgerald factor: a hitherto unrecognized coagulation factor. *Lancet* i, 949.

WERLE E. (1968) Contribution to the biochemistry of Trasylol. In: *New Aspects of Trasylol Therapy. The Clinical Significance of the Vascular and Circulatory Action of Trasylol. Report on an International Symposium.* (Haberland G.L. and Matis P. eds.) pp. 51-62, F.K. Schattauer Verlag, Stuttgart.

WERLE E. (1971) Trasylol: a short survey of its history, biochemistry and activities. In: *New Aspects of Trasylol Therapy. Protease Inhibiton in Shock Therapy. Report on an International Symposium.* (Brendel W. and Haberland G.L., eds.) pp. 9-16, F.K. Schattauer Verlag, Stuttgart.

WILKENS H.J. STEGER R. and BACK N. (1975) Effects of the protease inhibitor Trasylol in acute coronary occlusion in the dog. In: *New Aspects of Trasylol Therapy. Experimental Myocardial Infarction. Report on an International Symposium.* (Cantin M., Haberland G.L., Schnells G. and Selye H., eds.) pp. 381-392, F.K. Schattauer Verlag, Stuttgart.

WUEPPER K.D. (1973) Prekallikrein deficiency in man. *Amer. J. Med.* 138, 1345.

# Report on epsilon aminocaproic acid (EACA) (6-aminohexanoic acid)[1]

## Chemistry

A non-physiological amino acid, related to lysine, which can be synthesized as a white crystalline material freely soluble in water and of molecular weight 131 (Okamoto and Hijikata, 1975).

$CH_2CH_2CH_2CH_2CH_2COOH$  
$|$  
$NH_2$

$CH_2CH_2CH_2CH_2\ CH_2COOH$  
$|\qquad\qquad\qquad |$  
$NH_2\qquad\qquad\quad NH_2$

EACA                                    LYSINE

## Theoretical mode of action as a haemostatic

EACA is a protease inhibitor with its greatest activity against plasminogen activators. When measured by standard clot systems, EACA at a concentration of $10^{-4}M$ is a competitive inhibitor of streptokinase (SK), urokinase (UK), tissue activators and the spontaneous activity found in blood (Alkjaersig et al., 1959; Ablondi et al., 1959). At higher concentrations, above $5 \times 10^{-2}$ M, EACA shows non-competitive inhibition of other proteolytic enzymes including plasmin, trypsin and pepsin. These properties have been related to the carbon chain length of the molecule and its terminal amino and carboxyl groups (Okamoto and Hijikata 1975). It has been suggested that EACA binds to and alters the conformation of plasminogen (Ablondi et al., 1959; Abiko et al., 1969; Brockway and Castellino, 1972). However, the undoubted overall inhibitory effect on fibrinolysis in standard clot systems remains unexplained since in purified systems analysed by sodium dodecyl sulphate gel electrophoresis concentrations of EACA up to $10^{-3}M$

1. Acikaprin®, Afibrin®, Amicar®, Capracid®, Capramol®, Caprocid®, Caprolest®, Caprolisin®, EACA-Roche®, Eacina®, Ecapron®, Epsikapron®, Epsilon-Tachostyptan®, Hemocaprol®.

actually accelerate the activation of plasminogen some 75-fold (Walther *et al.*, 1974). This acceleration is in the first stage of plasminogen activation, the cleavage of the pre-activation peptide from the $NH_2$-terminal end of native plasminogen ($NH_2$-terminal glutamic acid). The second stage of activation, cleavage of an arginyl-valyl bond to give the two-chain structure of plasmin, is not affected by EACA at this concentration. However, at concentrations above $10^{-2}M$ EACA inhibits both stages in these purified systems. Perhaps the inhibitory effect on standard clot systems of lower concentrations depends on the modification of the substrate fibrin (Ambrus *et al.*, 1968).

Tosyl arginyl methyl esterase activity generated in systems containing plasminogen either by SK or by UK is not affected by any concentration of EACA (Ambrus *et al.*, 1968; Abiko *et al.*, 1969). EACA above $10^{-4}M$ inhibits the activation of plasminogen by SK but not by UK when the plasmin generated is measured by the breakdown of a casein substrate (Ambrus *et al.*, 1968).

The haemostatic action of EACA is thought to depend upon its ability to inhibit fibrinolysis. With therapeutic doses, a concentration of approximately $10^{-3}M$ can be achieved in the blood and body fluids. There, inhibition of plasminogen activators may preserve fibrin in haemostatic plugs threatened by normal fibrinolytic activity. In certain circumstances this activity may even be increased locally or throughout the vascular system (Nilsson, 1975; Prentice, 1975).

The measurable effects of EACA on standard tests of *in vivo* fibrinolysis have been variably reported. Most agree that spontaneous fibrinolysis is still apparent in the dilute blood clot and euglobulin clot lysis times especially the latter since EACA is not precipitated (e.g. Gordon-Smith *et al.*, 1972). Beck *et al.* (1963) gave 10 g EACA i.v. in 1 h to normal adults and found that euglobulin lysis times were shorter, implying increased fibrinolysis, for 2 h after the infusion. The same authors also administered a 'titrated initial dose' of SK to normals. 10 g of EACA given before or after the SK did not change the measured effects of standard tests. The inhibition of *in vivo* fibrinolysis by EACA is therefore incomplete.

EACA has other ill-defined actions, which might relate to any possible haemostatic effect. Kinin release by protease is weakly inhibited (Back and Steger, 1968); the noradrenaline content of the hearts of rats, mice and dogs is reduced (Lippman and Wishnick, 1965) and myocardial contractibility in dogs is improved (Nolan *et al.*, 1968); certain allergic reactions are said to be blocked (Raab, 1968; Bennett and Ogston, 1973); C'1 esterase release may be inhibited (Frank *et al.*, 1972). No direct action on blood coagulation has been reported at therapeutic concentrations.

## Pharmacology

This has been investigated by McNicol *et al.* (1962) and by Andersson *et al.* (1968). Oral doses are rapidly absorbed giving peak plasma levels after 2 h. The drug becomes distributed throughout the body water; diffusion into cells may inhibit cellular uptake of lysine. EACA is excreted and concentrated in the urine in a chemically unchanged active form, the greater part of a dose being excreted within 12 h. This rapid excretion means that parenteral administration for systemic reasons should be by continuous infusion; plasma levels of $10^{-3}M$ in the average adult can also be maintained by oral doses of 4-6 g followed by 4 g every 4 h. However, less frequent doses are adequate for action in the renal tract, where EACA is concentrated.

## Toxicology and side effects

10-20% of patients show headache, nausea, diarrhoea, nasal stuffiness, or conjunctival suffusion. Less frequently there may be hypotension for some hours. Osmotic diuresis with 36 g daily may give electrolytic disturbances. Very high doses have produced subendocardial haemorrhage in dogs and monkeys (Lippman and Wishnick, 1965). The drug is said to be teratogenic in animals (Johnson *et al.*, 1962). Prolonged toxicity studies in animals have shown no ill-effects despite the likelihood of the incorporation of EACA in place of lysine in body proteins. However, widespread muscle necrosis developed during long-term EACA therapy for angioneurotic oedema in one patient (Korsan-Bengsten *et al.*, 1969), and muscle pains and weakness following EACA have been associated with increases in serum creatine phosphokinase and aldolase (Frank *et al.*, 1972).

The main, hypothetical, danger is that inhibition of fibrinolysis may predispose to thrombosis, or prevent normal lysis of preformed intravascular or extravascular fibrin. There are many isolated reports of arterial or venous thrombosis in association with EACA therapy, but in each case a disease known to predispose to the complication has also been present. Detailed studies using phlebography (Becker and Borgström, 1968) or $^{125}$I-fibrinogen uptake (Gordon-Smith et al., 1972) show no change in the incidence of venous thrombosis attributable to EACA after prostatectomy. In a double-blind multicentre study of 515 patients the mortality due to pulmonary embolism and myocardial infarction was comparable in control and EACA treated groups (Vinnicombe and Shuttleworth, 1966 a). There is thus no evidence that EACA predisposes to thrombosis.

On the other hand, there is no doubt that EACA can perpetuate existing fibrin deposits. Persistence of extravascular fibrin has been noted in the pleural cavity following cardiac surgery, with unlysable clots requiring pulmonary decortication (Ratnoff, 1969) and in the kidney causing complete loss of renal function (McNicol et al., 1961). However, an increased incidence of clot retention has not been reported after the use of EACA in association with prostatectomy or with EACA for haematuria in sickle cell disease (Immergut and Stevenson, 1965).

## Clinical studies

EACA has been advocated in hyperfibrinolytic states, either therapeutically induced or spontaneous. While logical in the former, no studies confirm this and rapid clearance of SK and UK make it unnecessary. There is no evidence that it reduces the anti-haemostatic effects of fibrinogen/fibrin degradation products. Doubt remains as to the relative importance of thrombin and plasmin in the production of fibrinogenopenia in the haemorrhagic 'defibrination syndrome'; EACA is as difficult to assess as heparin; there is no definitive study. A theoretical danger of intravascular thrombosis is supported by numerous reports of thrombosis with EACA treatment in conditions likely to be characterized by diffuse intravascular coagulation.

EACA is, however, a proven haemostatic agent in a limited number of conditions in which there is no evidence for an increase in systemic fibrinolysis, primary or secondary. While local fibrinolysis may be enhanced in some diseased tissues the incidence is difficult to evaluate; there seems no need to postulate any increase in view of the ubiquitous nature of fibrinolytic enzymes.

Selecting only prospective, randomized, controlled trials, in which the groups have been shown to correspond, where objective methods of assessment have been used, where careful statistical analysis supports the conclusion, and where trials have been conducted by several groups with no dissenting results, there is clear evidence that EACA is a haemostatic agent in three clinical situations: prostatectomy, menorrhagia, and for dental extraction in haemophilia. One double-blind trial which meets the other conditions showed reduced blood loss with EACA in adenotonsillectomy (Verstraete *et al.*, 1968).

*Prostatectomy.* Blood loss during transvesical or transurethral prostatectomy is not affected by EACA. In the immediate postoperative and succeeding periods, EACA in doses of 5 g i.v. 6 hourly for 60 hours (Sack *et al.*, 1962), 20 g i.v. over 13 to 30 hours (Lawrence *et al.*, 1966) or 6 g i.v. over 12 hours (Vinnicombe and Shuttleworth, 1966b) halved the measured blood loss and reduced the duration of bleeding without a significant increase in clot retention. After transurethral prostatectomy blood loss was at least halved by EACA 15 g in 10 hours (Madsen and Strauch, 1966), 60 g over 60 hours (Warren and Stanley, 1969) or 16 g over 12 hours (Smart *et al.*, 1974).
In the study by Lawrence *et al.*, (1966) there was no relation between blood loss and measured urinary UK activity. All reports use EACA before, during or just after operation as prophylaxis against bleeding; there have been no trials of the use of EACA once profuse secondary bleeding has occured. A general review of antifibrinolytic drugs in the treatment of urinary tract haemorrhage is given by Andersson (1972).

*Menorrhagia.* Using objective measurement of blood lost at menstruation, Nilsson and Rybo (1965) gave 18 g EACA p.o. for the first 3 days of a period, then 12, 9, 6 and 3 g daily to 37 patients in a double-blind cross-over study. This reduced blood loss from $127 \pm 22$ ml to $52 \pm 8$ ml ($p < 0.001$). Cross-over studies in women with an intrauterine contraceptive device also reduced menstrual losses by 50% when EACA 3 g q.d.s. during menstruation were given (Kasonde and Bonnar, 1975 a, b). EACA has also been compared favourably with other therapy for menorrhagia (Nilsson and Rybo, 1971). Full investigations should first exclude an underlying neoplasm.

*Dental extraction in haemophilia.* EACA reduces the amount of therapeutic coagulation-factor concentrates necessary to reduce intra-oral bleeding after tooth extraction in the inherited bleeding disorders including haemophilia and Christmas disease. EACA is given together with specific coagulation factor concentrate to increase the factor level to at least 50% of normal, before operation. EACA is given as 6 g orally q.d.s. for 7-10 days, including one dose i.v. within 2 h before the extraction (Walsh *et al.*, 1971). In this and other studies (Walsh *et al.*, 1975) it is noteworthy that the usual time of onset of bleeding in control patients was the third postoperative day, suggesting that it took that time for natural fibrinolysis to remove a clot formed at the original operation. It has been estimated that the need for factor VIII concentrates to cover dental extraction can be reduced from 11,062 units/patient to 717 units/patient. This may have importance for other types of surgery in the bleeding disorders. However, for operations in which the bleeding might be life-threatening or where wound disruption might have serious consequences, any formal trial which withheld therapy from controls would be difficult to justify and is probably unnecessary. There have been suggestions, but no proof, that EACA may reduce the incidence of spontaneous haemarthroses in haemophilia (Gordon *et al.*, 1965).

## Conclusions

There can be no doubt that EACA is an effective haemostatic when used to reduce menstrual blood loss, when given before prostatectomy to reduce blood loss after operation, and when given before dental extraction together with coagulation factor concentrates to a patient with a congenital bleeding disorder. Certainly in the latter case, the use of the drug is of considerable clinical importance and its use without formal trial should be considered for all operations in patients with congenital or acquired coagulation disorders. There is no evidence that EACA predisposes to thrombosis but it certainly perpetuates existing fibrin deposits. Its use is therefore contraindicated when there are blood clots in the body cavities and it should be used with caution, if at all, if there is bleeding into the renal pelvis. There are theoretical dangers in the use of EACA in any state likely to be associated with diffuse intravascular coagulation, where the increase in fibrinolysis may have an important compensatory effect. The proven haemostatic effect must therefore be set against these possible dangers and, although bleeding will often be reduced in amount, it is important to show that this provides real clinical benefit. In the future the action of EACA must be compared with other systemic amino acids of similar activity, such as tranexamic acid.

## REFERENCES

ABIKO Y., IWAMOTO M. and TOMIKAWA M. (1969) Plasminogen-plasmin system V. A stoichiometric equilibrium complex of plasminogen and a synthetic inhibitor. *Biochim. biophys. Acta (Amst.)* 185, 424.

ABLONDI F.B., HAGAN J.J., PHILIPS M. and DE RENZO E.C. (1959) Inhibition of plasmin, trypsin and streptokinase activated fibrinolytic system by epsilon-aminocaproic acid. *Arch. Biochem.* 82, 153.

ALKJAERSIG N., FLETCHER A.P. and SHERRY S. (1959) E-Aminocaproic acid: an inhibitor of plasminogen activation. *J. biol. Chem.* 234, 832.

AMBRUS C.M., AMBRUS J.L., LASSMAN H.B. and MINK I.B. (1968) Studies on the mechanism of action of inhibitors of the fibrinolysin system. *Ann. N. Y. Acad. Sci.* 146, 430.

ANDERSSON L., NILSSON I.M., COLLEEN S., GRANSTAND B. and MELANDER B. (1968) Role of urokinase and tissue activator in sustaining bleeding and the management thereof with EACA and AMCA. *Ann. N. Y. Acad. Sci.* 146, 642.

ANDERSSON L. (1972) Antifibrinolytic drugs in the treatment of urinary tract haemorrhage. *Progr. Surg. (Basel)* 10, 76.

BACK N. and STEGER R. (1968) Effect of inhibitors on kinin-releasing activity of proteases. *Fed. Proc.* 27, 96.

BECK E., SCHMUTZLER R. and DUCKERT F. (1963) Inhibition of fibrinolysis and fibrinogenolysis in man: comparison of E-aminocaproic acid and kallikrein inhibitor. *Thrombos. Diathes. haemorrh. (Stuttg.)* 10, 106.

BECKER J. and BORGSTROM S. (1968) Incidence of thrombosis associated with epsilon-aminocaproic acid administration and with combined epsilon-aminocaproic acid and subcutaneous heparin therapy. *Acta chir. scand.* 134, 343.

BENNETT B. and OGSTON D. (1973) Natural and drug-induced inhibition of fibrinolysis. *Clinics in Haematology* 2, 135.

BROCKWAY W.J. and CASTELLINO F.J. (1972) Measurement of the binding of antifibrinolytic amino acids to various plasminogens. *Arch. Biochem.* 151, 194.

FRANK M.M., SERGENT J.S., KANE M.A. and ALLING D.W. (1972) Epsilon aminocaproic acid therapy of hereditary angioneurotic edema. *New Engl. J. Med.* 286, 808.

GORDON A.M., McNICOL G.P., DUBBER A.H.C., McDONALD G.A. and DOUGLAS A.S. (1965) Clinical trial of epsilon-aminocaproic acid in severe haemophilia. *Brit. med. J.* i, 1632.

GORDON-SMITH I.C., HICKMAN J.A. and EL MASRI S.H. (1972) The effect of the fibrinolytic inhibitor epsilon-aminocaproic acid on the incidence of deep-vein thrombosis after prostatectomy. *Brit. J. Surg.* 59, 522.

IMMERGUT M.A. and STEVENSON T. (1965) The use of epsilon aminocaproic acid in the control of haematuria associated with haemoglobinopathies. *J. Urol. (Baltimore)* 93, 110.

JOHNSON A.L., SKOZA L. and CLAUS E. (1962) Observations on epsilon aminocaproic acid. *Thrombos. Diathes. haemorrh. (Stuttg.)* 7, 203.

KASONDE J.M. and BONNAR J. (1975a) Aminocaproic acid and menstrual loss in women using intrauterine devices. *Brit. Med. J.* iv, 17.

KASONDE J.M. and BONNAR J. (1975b) Effect of ethamsylate and aminocaproic acid on menstrual blood loss in women using intrauterine devices. *Brit. Med. J.* iv, 21.

KORSAN-BENGSTEN K., YSANDER L. and BLOHME G. (1969) Extensive muscle necrosis after long-term treatment with aminocaproic acid (EACA) in a case of hereditary periodic oedema. *Acta med. scand.* 185, 341.

LAWRENCE A.C.K., WARD-McQUAID J.N. and HOLDOM G.L. (1966) The effect of epsilon aminocaproic acid on the blood loss after retropubic prostatectomy. *Brit. J. Urol.* 38, 308.

LIPPMAN W. and WISHNICK M. (1965) Effects of the administration of epsilon aminocaproic acid on catecholamine and serotonin levels in the rat and dog. *J. Pharmacol. exp. Ther.* 150, 196.

MADSEN P.O. and STRAUCH A.E. (1966) The effect of aminocaproic acid on bleeding following transurethral prostatectomy. *J. Urol. (Baltimore)* 96, 255.

McNICOL G.P., FLETCHER A.P., ALKJAERSIG N. and SHERRY S. (1961) Use of epsilon aminocaproic acid a potent inhibitor of fibrinolytic activity in management of postoperative haematuria. *J. Urol. (Baltimore)* 86, 829.

McNICOL G.P., FLETCHER A.P., ALKJAERSIG N. and SHERRY S. (1962) The absorption, distribution and excretion of epsilon-aminocaproic acid following oral or intravenous administration to man. *J. Lab. clin. Med.* 59, 15.

NILSSON I.M. (1975) Local fibrinolysis as a mechanism for haemorrhage. *Thrombos. Diathes. haemorrh. (Stuttg.)* 34, 623.

NILSSON I.M., ANDERSSON L. and BJORKMAN S.E. (1966) Epsilon-aminocaproic acid (EACA) as a therapeutic agent. Based on 5 years clinical experience. *Acta med. scand.,* suppl. 448.

NILSSON L. and RYBO G. (1965) Treatment of menorrhagia with epsilon-aminocaproic acid. *Acta obstet. gynec. scand.* 44, 467.

NILSSON L. and RYBO G. (1971) Treatment of menorrhagia. *Amer. J. Obstet. Gynec.* 110, 713.

NOLAN S.P., DIXON S.H.Jr., BEHRENDT D.M. and MORROW A.G. (1968) The effects of epsilon-aminocaproic acid on ventricular performance and total peripheral vascular resistance. *Ann. Surg.* 167, 547.

OKAMOTO S. and HIJIKATA A. (1975) Rational approach to proteinase inhibitors. *Drug Design* 6, 143.

PRENTICE C.R.M. (1975) Indications for antifibrinolytic therapy. *Thrombos. Diathes. haemorrh. (Stuttg.)* 34, 634.

RAAB W. (1968) Influence of antifibrinolytic substances on allergic reactions. Experiments with E-aminocaproic acid and amino-methyl-cyclohexane-carbonic acid. *Experientia (Basel)* 24, 250.

RATNOFF O. (1969) Epsilon aminocaproic acid. A dangerous weapon. *New Engl. J. Med.* 280, 1124.

SACK E., SPAET T.H., GENTILE R.L. and HUDSON P.B. (1962) Reduction of postprostatec-tomy bleeding by epsilon-aminocaproic acid. *New. Engl. J. Med.* 266, 541.

SMART C.J., TURNBULL A.R. and JENKINS J.D. (1974) The use of frusemide and epsilon-aminocaproic acid in transurethral prostatectomy. *Brit. J. Urol.* 46, 521.

VERSTRAETE M., VERMYLEN J. and TYBERGHEIN J. (1968) Double-blind evaluation of the haemostatic effect of adrenochrome monosemicarbazone, conjugated oestrogens and epsilon aminocaproic acid after adenotonsillectomy. *Acta haemat. (Basel)* 40, 154.

VINNICOMBE J. and SHUTTLEWORTH K.E.D. (1966a) Aminocaproic acid in the control of haemorrhage after prostatectomy. Safety of aminocaproic acid. A controlled trial. *Lancet i,* 232.

VINNICOMBE J. and SHUTTLEWORTH K.E.D. (1966b) Aminocaproic acid in the control of haemorrhage after prostatectomy. A controlled trial. *Lancet i,* 230.

WALSH P.N., RIZZA C.R., MATTHEWS J.M., EIPE J., KERNOFF P.B.A., COLES M.D., BLOOM A.L., KAUFMAN B.M., BECK P., HANAN C.M. and BIGGS R. (1971) Epsilon-aminocaproic acid therapy for dental extractions in haemophilia and Christmas disease: a double-blind controlled trial. *Brit. J. Haemat.* 20, 463.

WALSH P.N., RIZZA C.R., EVANS B.E. and ALEDORT L.M. (1975) The therapeutic role of epsilon-aminocaproic acid (EACA) for dental extractions in haemophiliacs. *Ann. N. Y. Acad. Sci.* 290, 267.

WALTHER P.J., HILL R.L. and McKEE P.A. (1974) The importance of the preactivation peptide in the two-stage mechanism of human plasminogen activation. *J. biol. Chem.* 250, 5926.

WARREN J.W. Jr. and STANLEY K.E. Jr. (1969) New anti-hemorrhagic agent. Epsilon aminocaproic acid for control of hemorrhage after transurethral prostatic resection: a control study. *J. Kansas med. Soc.* 20, 173.

# Report on p-aminomethyl-benzoic acid [1]
# (PAMBA)

## Chemistry

PAMBA is p-aminomethyl-benzoic acid.

$$H_2N-CH_2 \text{—}\langle benzene \rangle\text{—}COOH \qquad \text{M.W. 151.2}$$

It is a colourless, odourless, microcrystalline powder with a faintly bitter taste. It dissolves slowly in cold water, but is easily soluble in water at 100°C (to 4%).

## Theoretical mode of action

PAMBA was first described in 1963 by Marckwardt who discovered its antifibrinolytic action. Characteristic for this drug is the 7 Å spacing between the $NH_2$ and COOH groups, just as in ε-aminocaproic acid (EACA). Comparison of EACA and PAMBA showed that the latter was about 3 times more active. This was true in a euglobulin lysis test, on fibrin plates and in a test for inhibition of the streptokinase-induced fibrinolytic activity. A direct antiplasmin activity was not detected by Andersson *et al.* (1971), but was, however, reported by Landmann (1967).

## Pharmacokinetics

PAMBA is readily absorbed within a maximum of 2-3 h after oral administration. Excretion is via the kidneys. 50% is excreted unchanged during the first 24 h; 25% in the first 3 h. 20% is excreted as acetyl PAMBA which has no antifibrinolytic action. The plasma half-life is 1 h.

1. Gumbix®, Styptosolut®

The distribution volume is 0.58 l/kg. Andersson *et al.* (1971) have claimed that an adequate antifibrinolytic effect would require 80% inhibition. This is reached at a plasma level of 25 µg/g.

PAMBA is not toxic. In mice the $LD_{50}$ was 2,700 mg/kg (intra-peritoneal). Wistar rats showed no effects with a dose of 2,500 mg/kg i.p.; and 250 mg/kg over a 6-week period produced no ill-effects.

## Efficacy in patients with a bleeding disorder

No controlled randomized or double-blind studies were carried out. The data are included in Table 1.

## Efficacy in patients without a bleeding disorder

The various clinical investigations carried out with PAMBA are summarized in Table 1. No controlled, randomized or double-blind study has been carried out, with one possible exception (Andersson *et al.*, 1971), but this investigation was not published in detail.

## Side effects

PAMBA is well tolerated. Nausea, vomiting, diarrhoea and vertigo are rare. Fluctuations in blood pressure, sometimes with increased pulse rate, were noted during and directly after injection.

## Recommended dose

PAMBA is marketed as Gumbix®. One tablet contains 100 mg PAMBA and one 5 ml ampoule contains 50 mg PAMBA.

The dose recommended by the manufacturer is 1-2 tablets, 3 times daily, or 1-3 ampoules administered slowly i.v. or i.m.

The maximum single dose is 1000 mg orally or 200 mg i.v. or i.m. The maximum daily dose is 2 g orally or 600 mg i.v. or i.m.

In view of the investigations of Andersson *et al.* (1971) and in comparison with the experience with tranexamic acid, this recommended dosage seems much too low. It would be interesting to know what the basis for this recommendation is.

Table 1. Clinical investigations on PAMBA.

| Reference | indication | administration | patient | control | random | blind | objective criteria |
|---|---|---|---|---|---|---|---|
| Boeminghaus (1972) | prostatectomy | local | – | – | – | – | ± |
| Frank and Limbacher (1974) | prostatectomy | i.v. | ± | + | – | – | – |
| Linz (1969) | hypermenorrhoea | p.o | – | – | – | – | – |
| Flähmig et al. (1965) | hypermenorrhoea | p.o./i.v. | – | – | – | – | – |
| Sundermann and Vogel (1965) | haematuria | p.o. | 2 case reports | + | – | + | ± |
| Hellinger (1967) | haematuria + prostate | p.o., i.v., i.m. | – | ± | – | – | –/± |
| Neef et al. (1967) | prostate | i.v./i.m. | – | + | – | – | + |
| Hoffmann et al. (1967) | essent. haematuria | p.o. | + | – | – | – | ±/+ |
| Vogel (1967) | thrombopenia | p.o. | – | – | – | – | + |
| Sundermann (1967) | case report | p.o. | + | – | – | – | – |
| Hellinger (1967) | case report | i.v. | + | – | – | – | ± |
| Flähmig et al. (1967) | menstruation | p.o./i.v. | ± | – | – | – | – |
| Sieg and Flähmig (1967) | solutio + toxicose | i.v. | ± | – | – | – | ± |
| Rothe (1967) | tooth extraction | local + i.v. | ++ | – | – | – | – |
| Nuernbergh (1967) | tonsillectomy | i.v. | 2 case reports | – | – | – | + |
| Hoffmann and Mey (1967) | miscellaneous | p.o. | – | – | – | – | – |
| Wessel (1967) | rheumatic disease | i.m. | polyarth. | – | – | – | + |
| Andersson et al. (1971) | hypermenorrhoea | p.o. | ± | + | + | ? | + |
| Mey et al. (1967) | haemorrh. diath. | p.o. | – | – | – | – | ± |
| Hellinger (1966) | haematuria | i.m. | – | – | – | – | – |
| Davidoff (1970) | dental surgery | p.o. | – | – | – | – | + |
| Sieg and Flähmig (1969) | pre-eclampsia | p.o. | – | – | – | – | – |
| | puerperal bleeding | i.v. | – | – | – | – | – |

## Conclusions

PAMBA is a potentially useful antifibrinolytic drug. It has a number of attractive properties (low toxicity, high efficacy) which could make it a valuable drug. No definite answer can be given yet about its clinical efficacy.

REFERENCES

ANDERSSON L., NILSSON I.M., LIEDBERG G., NILLSON L., RYBO G., ERIKSON O., GRANDSTRAND B. and MELANDER B. (1971) Vergleichende Untersuchungen von trans-4-(Aminomethyl)-cyclohexan-carbonsàure Aminocapronsàure und p-Aminomethylbenzoesäure. *Arzneimittel-Forsch.* 21, 424.
BOEMINGHAUS F. (1972) Intravesikale Applikation von Antifibrinolytika nach Eingriffen an der Prostata. *Z. Urol.* 10, 771.
DAVIDOFF S.M. (1970) Erfahrungen mit dem Antifibrinolytikum PAMBA in der Kiefer-Gesichts-Chirurgie. *Dtsch. Stomat.* 20, 391.
FLAHMIG M., SIEG U. and VOGEL G. (1965) Fibrinolytische Störungen im uterinen Blut und ihre Beeinflussbarkeit durch p-Aminomethylbenzoesäure (PAMBA). *Münch. med. Wschr.* 107, 2007.
FLAHMIG M., SIEG U. and VOGEL G. (1967) Das Bild der fibrinolytische Störung im uterinen Blut und die Beeinflussbarkeit durch PAMBA. *Folia Haemat. (Lpz.)* 87, 41.
FRANK W. and LIMBACHER G. (1974) Vergleichende Untersuchungen zweier Hämostyptica bei Prostatektomierten. *Urologe* 13, 27.
HELLINGER J. (1966) Die Bedeutung lokaler Fibrinolysesteigerungen bei der symptomatische Hämaturie und ihre Hemmung durch p-Aminomethylbenzoesaure. *Z. Urol.* 59, 633.
HELLINGER J. (1967) Fibrinolyseblutungen in der Chirurgie und ihre Behandlung mit p-Aminomethylbenzoesaure. *Folia Haemat. (Lpz.)* 87, 32.
HELLINGER J. (1967) Die Anwendung von PAMBA in der Urologie. *Folia Haemat. (Lpz.)* 88, 187.
HOFFMANN W. and MEY U. (1967) Fibrinolyseblutungen im Kindesalter und ihre Blutungen mit PAMBA. *Folia Haemat. (Lpz.)* 87, 88.
HOFFMANN W. et al. (1967) Die Behandlung essentieller und symptomatischer Hamaturien im Kindesalter mit Antifibrinolytika. *Folia Haemat. (Lpz.)* 88, 203.
LANDMANN H. (1967) Vergleichende Untersuchungen über Antifibrinolytika. *Folia Haemat. (Lpz.)* 87, 106.
LINZ O. (1969) Zur Therapie funktioneller pathologischer Üterusblutungen mit PAMBA-Tabletten. *Dtsch. Gesundh.-Wes.* 24, 921.
MEY U., SUNDERMAN A. and VOGEL G. (1967) Begleitfibrinolysen bei hämatologischen Erkrankungen und ihre Beeinflussung durch PAMBA. *Folia Haemat. (Lpz.)* 87, 80.
NEEF H., PREUSSER K.P. and ANGER G. (1967) PAMBA-Prophylaxe bei Prostatektomien. *Folia Haemat. (Lpz.)* 88, 197.
NUERNBERGH W. (1967) Hyperfibrinolytische Blutungen in der HNO-Heilkunde und ihre Behandlung mit PAMBA. *Folia Haemat. (Lpz.)* 87, 72.
ROTHE G. (1967) Anwendung von PAMBA in der Zahn- und Kieferheilkunde. *Folia Haemat. (Lpz.)* 87, 67.

SIEG U. and FLÄMIG M. (1967) Die Bedeutung der Fibrinolysesteigerung bei Nach-
geburtsblutungen und ihre Behandlung mit PAMBA. *Folia Haemat. (Lpz.)* 87, 51.
SIEG U. and FLÄHMIG M. (1969) Die fibrinolytische Aktivität des peripheren und des
uterinen Blutes und ihre Beeinflussung durch p-Aminomethylbenzoesäure (PAMBA)
bei Gestosen. *Zbl. Gynäk.* 51, 1662.
SUNDERMANN A. and VOGEL G. (1965) Hämaturie infolge gesteigerter Urokinase-Aktivität
ihre erfolgreiche Behandlung durch p-Aminomethylbenzoesäure (PAMBA). *Münch.
med. Wschr.* 107, 2003.
SUNDERMANN A. (1967) Klinische Erfahrungen mit p-Aminomethylbenzoesäure (PAMBA)
bei schweren akuten Fibrinolyseblutungen in der Inneren Medizin. *Folia Haemat.
(Lpz.)* 87, 22.
VOGEL G. (1967) Über den Einfluss von Proteaseninhibitoren und synthetischen Antifib-
rinolytika auf die Blutungszeit. *Folia Haemat. (Lpz.)* 88, 174.
WESSEL G. (1967) Zur Wirkung der Para-Aminomethylbenzoesäure (PAMBA) bei
Polyarthritis acuta und progressiva. *Folia Haemat. (Lpz.)* 87, 94.

# Report on tranexamic acid[1]

## Chemistry

Tranexamic acid is the trans-isomer of 4-aminomethylcyclohexane carboxylic acid. The initial investigations were made using a preparation containing a mixture of isomers, but it was subsequently found (Melander *et al.* 1964; Okamoto *et al.*, 1964) that only the trans-isomer is antifibrinolytically active.

Tranexamic acid is a synthetic amino acid with a molecular weight of 157. It is a white crystalline substance, freely soluble in water, acids and alkalis. The chemical configuration of tranexamic acid has been determined (Groth, 1968; Kadoya *et al.*, 1966).

## Theoretical mode of action

*In vitro* the most striking action of tranexamic acid is inhibition of plasminogen activation (Andersson *et al.*, 1965; Dubber *et al.*, 1965), at concentrations as low as $10^{-6}$ M. At high concentrations, tranexamic acid also inhibits trypsinogen activation by enterokinase, and trypsin and pepsin activity. Inhibition of plasmin is weak.

Tranexamic acid is a competitive inhibitor of plasminogen activation (Dubber *et al.*, 1965; Maki and Beller, 1966) and at higher concentrations a non-competitive inhibitor of plasmin; its mode of action is therefore very similar to that of ε-aminocaproic acid.

Direct comparison of the potencies of ε-aminocaproic acid and tranexamic acid have given results which have varied substantially according to the test systems used, but figures varying from 6 to 100 times more potency with tranexamic acid have been reported (Andersson *et al.*, 1965; Andersson *et al.*, 1968; Dubber *et al.*, 1964; Okamoto *et al.*,

1. Anvitoff®, Cyklokapron®, Exacyl®, Frénolyse®, Ugurol®.

1964); in fibrinolytic test systems, an overall figure of a 10-fold increment in potency seem to be the consensus.

## Pharmacokinetics

In man, after intravenous administration of 10 mg/kg body weight, about 30% of the administered dose is recovered in the urine during the first hour after administration; a total of about 55% is recovered during the first three hours and about 90% after 24 hours (Andersson et al., 1965, 1968).

After oral doses of 10-15 mg/kg, the amounts recovered in the urine after 1 hour, 3 hours and 24 hours are 1%, 13% and 39% respectively. Intravenous administration of 10 mg/kg of tranexamic acid gave plasma concentrations of 18.3, 9.6 and 5 µg/ml 1,3 and 5 hours after injection. The biological half life has been reported to be 80 minutes (Kaller, 1967).

Tranexamic acid inhibits fibrinolytic activity in the urine (Andersson et al., 1968). After an oral dose of 10 mg/kg there was substantial inhibition of urinary fibrinolytic activity for at least 24 hours.

Tranexamic acid crosses the placenta (Kullander and Nilsson, 1970).

## Toxicology

*Acute toxicity.* Manufacturer's data (AB Kabi) suggests that tranexamic acid has a low acute toxicity; for example the $LD_{50}$ for mice is 12,500 mg/kg after oral and 1,300 mg/kg after intravenous administration.

*Chronic toxicity.* In teratogenic studies in rats, rabbits and mice with doses up to 5,000 mg/kg per day no fetal abnormalities were found (Melander et al., 1965). Dogs fed 220 mg of tranexamic acid/kg body weight daily for 2 weeks showed no microscopic evidence of fibrin deposition in numerous body tissues (Steenblock and Celander, 1968).

*Retinal changes.* In dogs, retinal changes have been reported following the oral administration over a period of a year of doses approximately 7 times higher than the maximum recommended for man per kilogram body weight per day. Intravenous doses approximately 18 times the maximum recommended for man per kilogram per day produced retinal damage in one dog over seven days. Such changes were not observed in dogs receiving orally approximately 3.5 times the maximum recommended dose for man per kilogram body weight per day for a year nor in monkeys receiving approximately 18 times the maximum recommended dose for man per kilogram per day intravenously for 1 or 2 weeks. No retinal changes have been found in patients receiving tranexamic acid over periods ranging from several weeks to nine years (AB Kabi).

*Liver tumours.* In one strain of rats receiving oral doses approximately 27 times higher than the maximum dose recommended per kilogram per day for man, adenomas and adenocarcinomas of the liver have been demonstrated after the administration of tranexamic acid for a period of 22 months but not after 12 months. Such tumours did not occur in rats after oral administration of doses approximately 6 times higher than the maximum recommended for man (AB Kabi). In another strain of rats receiving the same doses for a period of 2 years no liver tumours were demonstrated. Tranexamic acid has no mutagenic effect in a variety of test systems.

*Predisposition to thrombosis.* Therapy with fibrinolytic inhibitors carries a theoretical risk of an increased tendency to thrombosis, and extravascular blood clots formed when the inhibitor is in the circulation may be resistant to physiological fibrinolysis. Recently Rydin and Lundberg (1976) have reported two patients receiving tranexamic acid for the control of menorrhagia, and Davies and Howell have reported one patient with hereditary angio-oedema being treated with tranexamic acid, who developed intracranial arterial thrombosis. The association of the tranexamic acid therapy with the intracranial lesions may have been fortuitous and further observations are needed to assess the reality of this potential hazard.

### Clinical efficacy in patients with a bleeding disorder

*Haemophilia and Christmas disease.*

(1) *Long-term prophylactic administration.* One well designed long-term study failed to show benefit (Bennett *et al.*, 1973) and another trial (Gebauer and Heigel, 1969) reported benefit on an anecdotal basis.

However Rainsford *et al.*, (1973) in a double-blind cross-over study in haemophilia found a reduction in spontaneous bleeding episodes, significant at the 5% level, with tranexamic acid 3 g per day. Further work is needed.

(2) *Tooth extraction.* Forbes *et al.* (1972) in a prospective randomized double-blind study found that tranexamic acid, 1 g three times a day for five days, given in conjunction with factor VII or IX significantly reduced blood loss and transfusion requirements after dental extraction in patients with haemophilia and Christmas disease. Björlin and Nilsson (1973) also found apparently good results with tranexamic acid in tooth extraction with haemophilia and Christmas disease in an uncontrolled trial.

*Generalized haemostatic failure due to other causes.* No data are available from prospective controlled studies with random allocation.

## Clinical efficacy in individuals without a generalized bleeding disorder

*Menorrhagia.* Nilsson and Rybo (1967) have demonstrated in a double-blind study with random allocation that menstrual blood loss is significantly reduced by tranexamic acid, the effect being greater with 6 g per day than with 3 g per day though significant at both dosage levels. With 3 g of tranexamic acid per day, a reduction in menorrhagia has also been seen by Vermylen *et al.* (1968) again in a double-blind trial with random allocation. Callender *et al.* (1970) also found a significant reduction in menorrhagia with tranexamic acid, 1 g 4 times a day; in this study menstrual blood loss was quantitated by means of radioactive iron and a total body counter.

*Menorrhagia following the insertion of a contraceptive intrauterine device (IUD).* Weström and Bengtsson (1970) in a well designed controlled trial with random allocation have demonstrated that 6 g of tranexamic acid daily reduced the uterine blood loss after the insertion of an IUD from 82.7% to 11.5%; this difference is highly significant.

*Bleeding after gynaecological surgery.* Rybo and Westerberg (1972) in a randomized double-blind trial found that 4.5 g of tranexamic acid daily reduced by an average of 70% the bleeding after cervical conization.

*Urinary tract bleeding.* Hedlund (1969) in a random double-blind trial of patients undergoing prostatectomy found that tranexamic acid in a dose of 12 g or 6 g during the 4 days immediately preceeding and following prostatectomy significantly reduced urinary blood loss. Rö *et al.* (1970) in a random study of 22 patients having reimplantation of ureters found a significant reduction in bleeding in the tranexamic acid treated group (15 mg/kg body weight orally on the day before operation; 10 mg/kg body weight intravenously immediately before operation and again in the evening; and for 7 days after operation 15 mg/kg body weight given twice daily). However, six of the ten patients treated with tranexamic acid had large clots in the urinary bladder.

*Acute upper alimentary bleeding.* Cormack *et al.* (1973), in a controlled trial of tranexamic acid, 1.5 g three times a day, in patients with acute upper gastrointestinal bleeding distal to the gastro-oesophageal junction, and not apparently due to hiatus hernia or oesophageal varicies, found that treatment «failed» in 7 of 62 patients given tranexamic acid and in 17 of 63 control patients. The criteria of success or failure were «continued bleeding, the need for further blood transfusion, and surgery». The weaknesses in the trial include the failure to carry out gastroscopy and lack of objective criteria of blood loss. A further study of tranexamic acid in upper gastrointestinal bleeding is indicated.

*Epistaxis.* In a controlled double-blind trial of patients with recurring epistaxis, Petruson (1974) compared tranexamic acid and placebo. Patients were graded on a «point scale» according to the severity and number of bleeds. The points were determined by the author during the day, but at night by the emergency doctor in the Ear, Nose and Throat Department. There was no objective measurement of blood loss and in particular swallowed blood was not determined. Small local bleedings when tampons were removed were not recorded. In this trial bleeding was less frequent and less severe in patients given tranexamic acid, and the time spent in hospital was significantly shorter. A further study with objective criteria is indicated.

*Bleeding following ear, nose and throat surgery.* Verstraete *et al.* (1977) have compared tranexamic acid and placebo in patients undergoing adenotonsillectomy. Blood loss was measured as haemoglobin eluted from tampons, towels, gowns and bed linen and all ejected or aspirated blood was also measured. However, swallowed blood was not measured. The authors unfortunately failed to quote exact details of the measured blood loss which they record in terms of being less or more than 5 mg per kg body weight, but on this basis, and excluding blood loss in the stools, there was significantly less bleeding with tranexamic acid than placebo. Again, a further study with adequate estimation of blood loss, perhaps with radiochromium labelling of the red cells, is indicated.

## Side effects

Manufacturer's data (AB Kabi) report in a few cases gastrointestinal side effects such as nausea and diarrhoea. The frequency of these has been found to be lower than with aminocaproic acid however (Gebauer and Heigel, 1969; Weström and Bengtsson, 1970; Gibbs and Corkhill, 1971). Occasionally, orthostatic reactions have been reported. Pain over the kidneys and obstruction of urine flow from the kidney has been found occasionally in haemophiliacs treated for massive haematuria. Clot retention in the urinary bladder, kidney and ureter in patients with urinary tract bleeding has been reported (Gebauer and Heigel, 1969).

## Administration and dosage

Tranexamic acid can be given by intravenous injection or by mouth. When given by injection the dose should be given slowly over a period of at least 5 minutes.

For prostatectomy the suggested dosage is 0.5 g intravenously 2 to 3 times daily for three days; for menorrhagia 1-1.5 g 3 to 4 times daily for three to four days; for dental surgery in haemophilia, 25 mg/kg body weight given by mouth 3 to 4 times daily for six to eight days, together with a suitable source of factor VIII or factor IX before operation.

## Conclusions

The established and proved clinical situations in which tranexamic acid is effective are:
(1) Menorrhagia - reducing this may be important as loss is recurring.

(2) Increased bleeding after the insertion of an IUD.

(3) Perhaps some gynaecological operations.

(4) Bleeding after urinary tract surgery.

(5) Given to reduce bleeding at the time of tooth extraction in patients with haemophilia and Christmas disease.

At the present time other indications for tranexamic acid (e.g. long term prophylactic therapy in haemophilia; subarachnoid haemorrhage; defibrination syndrome) are not adequately supported by well designed prospective double-blind controlled trials.

## REFERENCES

ANDERSSON L., NILSSON I. M., NILEHN J. E., HEDNER U., GRANSTRAND B., and MELANDER B. (1965) Experimental and clinical studies on AMCA, the antifibrinolytically active isomer of p-aminomethyl cyclohexanecarboxylic acid. *Scand. J. Haemat.* 2, 230.

ANDERSSON L., NILSSON I. M., COLLEEN S., GRANSTRAND B. and MELANDER B. (1968) Role of urokinase and tissue activators in sustaining bleeding and the management thereof with EACA and AMCA. *Ann. N.Y. Acad. Sci.* 146, 642.

BENNETT A. E., INGRAM G. I. C. and INGLISH P. J. (1973) Antifibrinolytic treatment in haemophilia: a controlled trial of prophylaxis with tranexamic acid. *Brit. J. Haemat.* 24, 83.

BJORLIN G. and NILSSON I. M. (1973) Tooth extractions in hemophiliacs after administration of a single dose of factor VIII or factor IX concentrate supplemented with AMCA. *Oral. Surg.* 36, 482.

CALLENDER S. T., WARNER G. T. and COPE E. (1970) Treatment of menorrhagia with tranexamic acid. A double-blind trial. *Brit. med. J.* iv, 214.

CORMACK F., JAEHER A. J., CHAKRABARTI R. R. and FEARNLEY G. R. (1973) Tranexamic acid in upper gastrointestinal haemorrhage. *Lancet* i, 1207.

DAVIES D. and HOWELL D. A. (1977) Tranexamic acid and arterial thrombosis. *Lancet* i, 49.

DUBBER A. H. C., McNICOL G. P., DOUGLAS A. S. and MELANDER B. (1964) Some properties of the antifibrinolytically active isomer of aminomethylcyclohexane carboxylic acid. *Lancet* ii, 1317.

DUBBER A. H. C., McNICOL G. P. and DOUGLAS A. S. (1965) Aminomethylcyclohexane carboxylic acid (AMCA), a new synthetic fibrinolytic inhibitor. *Brit. J. Haemat.* 11, 237.

FORBES C. D., BARR R. D., REID G., THOMSON C., PRENTICE C. R., McNICOL G. P. and DOUGLAS A. S. (1972) Tranexamic acid in control of hemorrhage after dental extraction in haemophilia and Christmas disease. *Brit. med. J.* ii, 311.

GEBAUER D. and HEIGEL K. (1969) Therapeutische Beeinflussung der Hämophilie durch AMCHA. *Med. Klin.* 64, 378.

GIBBS J. R. and CORKILL A. G. L. (1971) Use of an anti-fibrinolytic agent (tranexamic acid) in the management of ruptured intracranial aneurysms. *Postgrad. med. J.* 47, 199.

GROTH P. (1968) Crystal structure of the trans form of 1,4-aminomethylcyclohexanecarboxylic acid. *Acta chem. scand.* 22, 143.

HEDLUND P. O. (1969) Antifibrinolytic therapy with Cyclokapron in connection with prostatectomy. A double-blind study. *Scand. J. Urol. Nephrol.* 3, 177.

KADOYA S., HANAZAKI F. and IITAKA Y. (1966) The crystal structures of trans- and cis-4-aminomethylcyclohexane-1-carboxylic acid hydrohalides. *Acta Cryst.* 21, 38.

KALLER H. (1967) Enterale Resorption, Verteilung und Elimination von 4-Aminomethylcyclohexancarbonsäure (AMCHA) und ε-Aminocapronsäure (ACS) beim Menschen. *Naunyn Schmiedeberg's Arch. Pharmak. exp. Pathol.* 256, 160.

KULLANDER S. and NILSSON I. M. (1970) Human placental transfer of an antifibrinolytic agent (AMCA). *Acta obstet. gynecol. scand.* 49, 241.

MAKI M. and BELLER F. K. (1966) Comparative studies of fibrinolytic inhibitors in vitro. *Thrombos. Diathes. haemorrh. (Stuttg.)* 16, 668.

MELANDER B., GLINIECKI G., GRANSTRAND B. and HANSHOFF G. (1964) Experimental studies on the antifibrinolytic activity of AMCHA (Abstr. G 68), X Congr. Int. Soc. Haemat., Stockholm.

MELANDER B., GLINIECKI G., GRANSTRAND B. and HANSHOFF G. (1965) Biochemistry and toxicology of aminokapron; the antifibrinolytically active isomer of AMCHA. *Acta pharmacol. (Kbh.)* 22, 340.

NILSSON L. and RYBO G. (1967) Treatment of menorrhagia with epsilon aminocaproic acid. *Acta obstet. gynecol. scand.* 46, 572.

OKAMOTO S., KINJO K., OSHIBA S., MANGYO M., SHIMIZU M., SATO S. and OKAMOTO U. (1964) Behavior of tissue activators and the action of a series of potent inhibitors of fibrinolysis (Abstr. G 65). X Congr. Int. Soc. Haemat., Stockholm.

PETRUSON B. (1974) *Acta Otolaryng.*, suppl. 317

RAINSFORD S. G., JOAHAR A. J. and HALL A. (1973) Tranexamic acid in the control of spontaneous bleeding in severe haemophilia. *Thrombos Diathes. haemorrh. (Stuttg.)* 30, 272.

RÒ J. S., KNUTRO O. and STORMORKEN H. (1970) Antifibrinolytic treatment with tranexamic acid (AMCA) in pediatric urinary tract surgery. *J. pediat. Surg.* 5, 315.

RYBO G. and WESTERBERG H. (1972) The effect of tranexamic acid (AMCA) in postoperative bleeding after conization. *Acta obstet. gynecol. scand.* 51, 347.

RYDIN E. and LUNDBERG P. O. (1976) Tranexamic acid and intracranial thrombosis. *Lancet* ii, 49.

STEENBLOCK D. A. and CELANDER D. R. (1968) A light and electron microscopic study of arteries and other tissues from dogs subjected to chronic fibrinolytic inhibition with AMCHA. *Vasc. Surg.* 2, 149.

VERMYLEN J., VERHAEGEN-DECLERCQ M. L., VERSTRAETE M. and FIERENS F. (1968) A double-blind study of the effect of tranexamic acid in essential menorrhagia. *Thrombos. Diathes. haemorrh. (Stuttg.)* 20, 584.

VERSTRAETE M., TYBERGHEIN J., DE GREEF Y., DAEMS L. and VAN HOOF A. (1977) Double-blind trials with ethamsylate, batroxobin or tranexamic acid on blood loss after adenotonsillectomy. *Acta clin. belg.* 32, 136.

WESTROM L. and BENGTSSON L. P. (1970) Effect of tranexamic acid (AMCA) in menorrhagia with intrauterine contraceptive devices. A double-blind study. *J. Reprod. Med.* 5, 154.

# Comments by the manufacturer of Cyklokapron®

**by H. Kjellman, Kabi AB, Stockholm**

Studies in man have demonstrated that after intravenous administration of a single dose of 10-15 mg of tranexamic acid/kg body weight, the plasma concentration curve shows three monoexponential decays: the first is a very rapid one, the second has a half-life of 1.3-2.0 hours and the third has a half-life of 9-18 hours. About half of the dose is recovered in the urine during the first 3-4 hours, 90-95% within 24 hours and 95-99% between 48 and 72 hours, as unchanged tranexamic acid (Eriksson *et al.*, 1974; Pilbrant *et al.*, 1976). The uncorrected plasma clearance rate is 110-115 ml/min which, corrected for an average plasma protein binding of 15%, approximately equals glomerular filtration. After intravenous administration of 10 mg/kg body weight, plasma concentrations of 18, 10 and 5 mg/l were achieved 1, 3 and 5 hours after the injection (Kaller 1967). When 15 mg/kg body weight was given intravenously the plasma levels were 30, 13 and 0.4 mg/l 1, 3 and 24 hours after the injection (Pilbrant *et al.*, 1976).

After oral doses of 0.5 g and 2.0 g of tranexamic acid to fasting adult volunteers a peak plasma concentration was obtained within 2-4 hours. After an oral dose of 0.5 g of tranexamic acid plasma peak levels of 3.5 to 7.0 mg/l were obtained and after a dose of 2.0 g peak levels of 11.9 to 15.6 mg/l. A mean of 37% of the dose was recovered in the urine 72 hours after the administration. The uncorrected renal clearance rate was 105-130 ml/min.

Intravenous administration of 10 mg/kg body weight to patients with renal diseases showed that the biological half-life of tranexamic acid increased with decreased renal function. A decreased frequency of doses based on the patient's serum creatinine values has been recommended (Pilbrant *et al.*, 1976).

| Serum creatinine | Dose i.v. | Dose frequency |
|---|---|---|
| <133 mmol/l | 10 mg/kg | 2-4 times daily |
| 134-265 mmol/l | 10 mg/kg | every 12th hour |
| 266-442 mmol/l | 10 mg/kg | every 24th hour |
| >442 mmol/l | 10 mg/kg | every 48th hour |

REFERENCES

ERIKSSON O., KJELLMAN H., PILBRANT Å. and SCHANNONG M. (1974) Pharmakokinetics of tranexamic acid after intravenous administration to normal volunteers. *Europ. J. clin. Pharmacol.* 7, 375.

KALLER H. (1967) Enterale Resorption, Verteilung und Elimination von 4-Aminomethyl-cyclohexanecarbonsäure (AMCHA) und ε-Aminocapronsäure (ACS) beim Menschen. *Naunyn-Schmiedeberg's Arch. Pharmak. exp. Path.* 256, 160.

PILBRANT Å., ANDERSSON L., ERIKSSON O., KJELLMAN H., SCHANNONG M. and WIDLUND L. (1976) Tranexamsyra. Farmakokinetik hos friska och njurinsufficienta försökspersoner. Report presented at the Annual General Meeting of the Swedish Society of Medical Sciences, Stockholm.

# Haemostatic agents for topical use

Several substances have been proposed as haemostatics for local use, mainly to reduce capillary bleeding; they will not effectively impede bleeding from arteries or veins when there is appreciable intravascular pressure. A logical topical haemostatic application is the use of sterile human plasma or human fibrinogen sprayed with human thrombin during surgery to create a film of fibrin or a clot *in situ*.

Most of the haemostatic agents for local use are marketed as preparations which are absorbed from the site of application after varying periods of time.

**Purified thrombin**[1] can be used as a topical haemostatic either in a diluted solution (100 to 1000 NIH units/ml) or as a lyophilized powder. Thrombin will control capillary bleeding and promote adhesion of tissue surfaces e.g. fixation of tissue transplants or skin grafts. Bovine thrombin is usually used as, despite its origin, antigenicity is rare when it is employed topically. The usual content of a vial is 1000, 5,000 or 10,000 NIH units (one unit is that amount of thrombin required to clot 1 ml of standard fibrinogen solution in 15 seconds at 28°C). A thrombin solution can be sprayed with a syringe and a fine needle or can be used in conjunction with absorbable gelatin sponges. For many years a weak thrombin preparation prepared from rabbit blood has been used in America[2]. A thrombin solution can also be taken by mouth in cases of gastrointestinal bleeding provided its destruction is prevented by dissolving it in a phosphate buffer.

**Some snake venoms**[3] have a thrombin-like action as they can coagulate fibrinogen directly. The fibrin formed is, however, chemically different (only fibrinopeptide A is split off) from· thrombin-generated

1. Thrombase® (I.S.H.: Paris), Thrombin Topical® (Parke-Davis: Detroit), Thrombo-Tuffon® (Ligner and Fisher: Bühl, Baden), Topostasin® (Hoffmann-La Roche: Basle).
2. Hemostatic Rabbit Globulin of Parfentjev®
3. Botropase® (Ravizza: Muggiò, Milan), Reptilase® (Pentapharm: Basle), Stypven® (Wellcome: Beckenham).

fibrin (fibrinopeptide A and B are split off) and the clot formed does not completely resemble a normal clot.

**Purified extracts of viper venoms** such as Russell's Viper Venom are prepared as a dry powder; when reconstituted with water in a dilute solution (1/10,000), this substance acts as a powerful thromboplastin and rapidly activates prothrombin. Its action is even faster in the presence of lipids and supercedes that of the previously used tissue thromboplastin suspensions, which were acetone extracts of rabbit brain or lung tissue. The latter materials had the advantage of being harmless, but were almost inactive as topical haemostatics.

The venoms prepared from other snakes such as the Australian tiger snake and the fer-de-lance have also been used as local haemostatics.

Absorbable sponges of **skin gelatin**[4] are sterile, water insoluble, foamy materials which are usually moistened with saline or soaked in a thrombin solution before use. Gelatin sponges do not have the disadvantage of conventional cotton wool, namely the frequent occurrence of re-bleeding when the dressing is removed. Most of the gelatin sponges are completely absorbed in 4 to 6 weeks and may therefore be left in place after closure of the wound. Gelatin is easily destroyed if an inflammatory reaction accurs.

**Methyl cellulose**[5] is the water soluble, cotton-like methyl ether of cellulose. It is non-allergenic and capable of absorbing eight times its weight of fluid. It exerts its physical effect by mechanical pressure; with the absorption of fluid the material swells and compresses the bleeding capillaries. Once in position, the methyl cellulose pad attains the consistency of moist blotting paper; it can be removed easily and painlessly, leaving a dry wound.

**Oxidized cellulose**[6] is a specially treated form of surgical gauze or cotton which is made absorbable by oxidation with nitrogen dioxide. This spongy substance is said to promote coagulation by a reaction between

4. Gelfilm® (Upjohn: Kalamazoo, Mich.), Gelfoam® (Upjohn: Kalamazoo, Mich.) Sorbacel® (Hartmann: Heidenheim), Spongostan® (Ferrosan: Denmark), Sterispon® (Allen and Hanbury: London).
5. Cologel® (Lilly: Indianapolis), Hydrolose® (Upjohn: Kalamazoo, Mich.), Methocel® (Dow Chemical Co.: Indianapolis).
6. Hemo-Pak® (Johnson and Johnson: Slough), Oxycel® (Parke-Davis: Detroit), Sorbacel® (Wander: Berne), Surgicel® (Ethicon: Somerville, N.J.).

haemoglobin and cellulosic acid; it also provides a large surface area at the site of haemorrhage and the threads in the cotton provide reinforcement for the fibrin mesh. The absorption of oxidized cellulose may take 7 days to 7 weeks or longer. This material should not be used for implantation or packing in fractures because it interferes with bone regeneration and may cause cyst formation. Oxidized cellulose also inhibits epithelialization and is therefore not a good surface dressing. Oxidized regenerated cellulose[7], is prepared from alpha-cellulose and is also a polyanhydroglucuronic acid. This product does not dissolve in water, salt solution or plasma. Due to its negatively charged surface, clotting proceeds rapidly and the swollen material provides a matrix for fibrin, forming a partially artificial coagulum.

Because of its low pH, oxidized cellulose interferes with the activity of thrombin unless this enzyme is dissolved in a 0.5% sodium bicarbonate solution.

Oxidized cellulose does not cause local irritation.

**Calcium alginate**[8] is also absorbable and has the advantage that it is heat sterilizable.

**Microcrystalline collagen**[9] is a white, floury material prepared from bovine skin corium. The haemostatic activity of this material can be ascribed to an inherent tissue cohesive property of collagen itself, and to adhesion of platelets. This relatively new material is being used in cardiovascular surgery to arrest bleeding around arterial anastomoses. Several collagen preparations are made from pigskin and purified by proteolytic agents[10]. This material is easy to handle, non-immunogenic and completely absorbable. It has been shown to be an effective topical haemostatic agent in orthopaedic surgery, vascular surgery, in the treatment of burns and atonic skin ulcers, and in the treatment of liver rupture.

Another collagenous haemostatic is a dried, sterile foam of **native, equine collagen fibrils**[11] which is also absorbable and indicated in all surgical procedures as a specific local haemostatic when control of bleeding by surgical technique is ineffective or impractical.

7. Tabotamp® (Johnson and Johnson: Amersfort).
8. Hemalgan® (Delforge: Belgium)
9. MCC® (Avicon: Fort Worth, Tex.)
10. Collagen Fleece® (Pentapharm: Basle)
11. Tachotop® (Hormon-Chemie: Munich)

# A note on vitamin C and bioflavonoids in bleeding disorders

**Vitamin C** (ascorbic acid) has been used in diverse conditions often associated with scurvy, including haemorrhagic states. Although bleeding may occur in scurvy it is not pathognomonic for this disease. There is no evidence in man that ascorbic acid is of any value in bleeding disorders except when bleeding occurs strictly in association with scurvy, a very rare disease these days, or in exceptional clinical states associated with severe vitamin C deficiency (e.g. benzene intoxication).

**Bioflavonoids** are derivatives of flavone and are present in the water soluble extract of citrus fruits. The active material was initially named vitamin P because it decreased capillary permeability in experimental animals and in people with scurvy. Since the vitamin nature of the compound came into doubt, the term bioflavonoids has become the preferred one. The most commonly employed commercial preparations are rutin (e.g. hydroxyethylrutosides), hesperidin (present in citrin) and aesculin (the glucoside of 6,7-dihydrocoumarin), however more than 500 flavonoids have been identified and described.

These substances are said to decrease capillary fragility and permeability in experimental animals because they inhibit the auto-oxidation of adrenaline and of ascorbic acid and have a hyaluronidase inhibiting effect. They are also thought to catalyze the formation of capillary intracellular cement substance in the liver from ascorbic acid and a protein fraction. Their clinical usefulness is very much doubted in present overfed populations; moreover their intestinal absorption is very poor which casts serious doubt on many clinical studies. The data demonstrating that these agents can prevent bleeding after surgery are too fragmentary to warrant any positive recommendations for their use.

A haemostatic principle was considered to be present in the seed membrane of the groundnut *(Arachis hypogea)*; the isolated chromagen appears to be a flavonoid. There is also some suggestion that peanuts contain a choline dehydrogen citrate which has antifibrinolytic properties. Although some haemophilic patients had the impression that while consuming daily roasted peanuts or peanut butter the tenderness of a knee haemarthrosis subsided more rapidly, carefully controlled double-blind trials failed to demonstrate a subjective or objective difference during the administration of a peanut extract or a placebo.

One expects from a general haemostatic drug that when given therapeutically in well defined clinical situations, it causes a clinically relevant reduction of bleeding or when given prophylactically reduces a definable and significant haemorrhagic risk. None of the three substances discussed meets the expectations for a haemostatic drug as defined above and one wonders on which clinical grounds vitamin C and bioflavonoids are still being recommended as 'general haemostatic agents'.

# The following recommendations are made for trials set up to determine the clinical usefulness of systemic haemostatic agents

(1) Definition and appropriate selection of patients admitted to the trial: all inclusion and exclusion criteria used to select patients must be mentioned in detail. It is also important to know of certain associated diseases (e.g. hypertension, diabetes, etc.) which influence the intensity or duration of bleeding.

(2) Due recognition of the spontaneous arrest of bleeding. For this purpose it is essential to follow a contemporaneous control group. To ensure that the experimental drug and placebo are allocated to similar numbers of patients from each risk group, randomization of preselected patients must be used. When analysing the results one still has to demonstrate that the two groups were equal at the start with respect to variables which might have affected blood loss.

(3) To eliminate prejudicial circumstances and a subconscious bias on the part of the investigators a double-blind technique is essential. Neither the patients nor the people performing the trial should know which group is receiving the drug under test. The key to the code should become available to the investigators only after the trial is terminated and all the data have been recorded. It is also highly recommended that an independent third party should distribute the materials (similar presentation of placebo and experimental drugs) to the investigator, prepare the randomization tables, and collect and analyse the data which will subsequently be given to the interested parties after completion of the trial. This is so that neither the manufacturer nor the investigator knows the code before completion of the trial and analysis of the results.

(4) The operative technique for a given operation should remain the same throughout the entire trial and only a very small group of surgeons should preferably be involved. A uniform scheme of anaesthesia (type and dose of the anaesthetic) is to be used and the duration of the operation recorded.

(5) The actual quantity of blood lost during the operation and following it is to be measured and not estimated subjectively. In addition, the number of sponges used can help to confirm a clinical impression which is, however, still not hard data and should be substantiated by other evidence.

(6) The general management and treatment of the two groups are to be the same; great attention is to be paid to the blood transfusion requirements and serial haematocrit (haemoglobin) values. For a safer interpretation of the latter test, the volumes and timing of parenteral fluid administration are to be recorded.

(7) The possible side effects are to be noted and attention should be given to the incidence of thrombophlebitis, deep vein thrombosis and pulmonary embolism.

(8) A clear distinction between the therapeutic and prophylactic value of a drug is to be made. Appropriate trials must be devised to prove either the prophylactic or the therapeutic value of the new drug.

(9) Clinical trials performed with the experimental drug given simultaneously or subsequently by parenteral and oral routes do not prove the efficacy of oral treatment alone.

(10) In demonstrating the effectiveness of a general haemostatic agent the proponent is expected to define the clinical candidates and not to draw conclusions which may be valid for one subgroup of patients but which do not hold for a broader group. The main subgroups are:
a) individuals without a congenital or acquired bleeding disorder undergoing surgery with possible serious blood loss or where flooding the operative field with blood makes precise manipulation difficult.
b) women without a generalised bleeding disorder who have essential menorrhagia or metrorrhagia or bleeding related to an intra-uterine device.
c) patients with recurrent bleeding due to thrombocytopenia or constitutional functional platelet disorders.
d) patients with a lifelong or acquired coagulation disorder.
e) patients with a congenital or acquired vascular or connective tissue defect.

f) patients with generalized or local enhancement of the fibrinolytic system.

g) patients with diabetic retinopathy.

(11) A standard dose (in mg per kg body weight) for a given drug is to be studied, and it is also recommended that the possibly increased haemostatic properties (and drawbacks?) of tenfold this dose are also investigated; it is common experience that in certain dramatic conditions much higher doses of a given drug are administered in the hope of stopping life-threatening bleeding.

(12) Assessment of results: once included in the trial, patients may only be withdrawn on the basis of strict criteria for withdrawal which have been defined in advance. Nevertheless, the first analysis of the results should preferably be based on the intention of treatment, including the withdrawals. A clear and detailed statistical analysis of the results is to be presented.

The many variable factors affecting bleeding during and following surgical operations make it difficult to arrange standardized conditions. Also, accurate measurement of blood loss is a problem, but is, however, feasible, especially during the operation. Methods for measuring blood loss once the patient is outside the operating theatre are rather cumbersome.

During operation, and continuing for several days, the contents of all aspirators and urine collection bags and all washing fluids, can be collected; the blood from dressings, swabs, bandages and bedclothes can be washed out, a 5% sodium hydroxide solution added for 20 hours and the alkaline haematin concentration determined spectrophotometrically. The Perdometer (AB Lars Ljungberg, Stockholm) is a useful instrument for this procedure. Instead of determining alkaline haematin, the iron content can be measured. Another method is to weigh all used linen daily. Repeated determinations of the haemoglobin content and haematocrit value of venous blood samples drawn without contra-pressure can also give some information, but this technique used alone is not sufficient to provide hard data on blood loss. Parenteral fluid, plasma expander and blood requirements should, of course, be noted.

During and after transurethral resection of the prostate, bladder washings can be collected in a graduated vessel and the blood loss estimated colorimetrically by the acid haematin method.

In trials quantitating menstrual blood loss, all used sanitary towels or tampons can be placed in a plastic bag containing a trioxymethylene tablet, and this bag sent to the laboratory for determination of the haematin content as described above. About 2-4 µCi [$^{39}$Fe] ferric citrate is given intravenously, and two weeks later the total body count is measured and taken as baseline value. Thereafter each patient reports for a total body count at two-weekly intervals, and the radioactivity on each occasion is compared to the previous count. The blood loss between visits is estimated from the decrease in radioactivity, compensated for radioactive decay.

After dental extraction a similar method can be applied, or blood loss can be measured with $^{51}$Cr-labelled red cells. This entails collection of oral secretions and faeces over 24-hour periods for five days. It is advisable to give the patient a purgative on day four. There is, of course, no physiological evidence that bleeding and clotting times are in themselves influenced by the number of teeth extracted. Nevertheless it should be realised that the greater the number of teeth removed, the greater the surface area of the mouth covered by blood clots, which in turn increases the likelihood of tongue and cheek action dislodging the forming clots and so causing bleeding.

In gastrointestinal haemorrhage, blood loss in the stools can be measured with the $^{51}$Cr-labelled red cells method.

For the evaluation of blood loss in patients with recurrent epistaxis, the amount of blood on collected linen can be measured, but this method does not allow the determination of swallowed blood.

Capillary fragility can be measured with the angiosterrometer of Parrot or the capillodynamometer of Lavollay.

It is known that the activation of factor XII triggers off the long process of coagulation, and that, amongst other things, the altered surface of aggregated platelets provides the necessary site for activation of factor XII. If a substance were found which influenced the activity of factor XII then haemostasis at a local level might be expected. However, many results cast doubt on the idea that accelerated clotting results in a proportional reduction of bleeding and oozing.

For many years the prevailing opinion has been that mild haemostatics act at the capillary level, either on the intrinsic clotting mechanism or on capillary motility, diameter, fragility or permeability. It was assumed that the pressure and structural characteristics of larger vessels made them insufficiently responsive to these drugs. Consequently, the search for new haemostatic drugs was directed towards agents which acted on capillaries and minute vessels. Usually measurement of the bleeding time is one of the main tests employed in screening new substances and evaluating their clinical effects in man. It is important to standardize the test very rigidly and to accept only a mean bleeding time which is the average value of a statistically sufficient number of individual bleeding times measured under standardized conditions. In general, however, no therapeutic prediction can be made from a reduction in bleeding time when a drug is aimed at reducing spontaneous or surgically-induced bleeding. For this evaluation, only well planned and executed double-blind clinical trials with measured blood loss can determine the prophylactic or therapeutic efficacy of a given substance.

# Conclusions on the clinical efficiency of general haemostatic drugs

Medical journals are littered with promises of successful general haemostatic drugs and every year a new drug is offered which is better than the last and free from side effects. Most of the enthusiastic proponents have ignored the occurrence of spontaneous arrest of bleeding in individuals without a major bleeding disorder. The advent of an effective 'general' haemostatic drug for systemic use would, however, be greatly welcomed for the treatment of excessive bleeding in patients for whom specific treatment is not available. Indeed, in patients with a known bleeding disorder specific treatment is usually provided by substitution of the missing or defective coagulation component or correction of the haemostatic defect. There is, however, no point in overdosage with e.g. vitamin K or heparin antagonists in a vain attempt to correct the original disorder. Valuable drugs such as vitamin K are also often misused in patients with a normal prothrombin time, since no pharmacological effect can be expected.

Whenever possible the arrest of bleeding should also be tackled by local treatment as it is unlikely that normal haemostasis can be improved.

Although hypercoagulability and states of hypercoagulation can be induced by some 'haemostatic drugs', it is still not clearly established that low-grade 'coagulation' is associated with accelerated haemostsis and could *per se* reduce bleeding in surgical patients with a normal haemostatic balance, or prevent spontaneous bleeding in patients with a haemostatic defect.

In a limited number of clinical conditions without apparent surgical or haematological cause for the abnormal bleeding and in patients with various haemorrhagic diseases, clinical evidence begins to emerge that a few general haemostatic drugs can reduce blood loss. Double-blind trials with quantitation of blood loss have shown that the antifibrinolytic agents epsilon aminocaproic acid and tranexamic acid are clinically effective after prostatectomy, adenotonsillectomy, tooth extraction (even in haemophiliacs), in essential menorrhagia and after the insertion of an

IUD. Ethamsylate seems to be an effective haemostatic drug in primary menorrhagia. It is possible that with some of the other general haemostatic drugs discussed in this book, the bleeding intensity can also be reduced but this has not yet been definitely proved by means of adequate trials.

# Haemostatic drugs mentioned in the text

| | |
|---|---|
| Acikaprin® | Polfa (Warsaw) |
| Adona AC-17® | Tanabe Seiyoku (Osaka) |
| Adrenosem® | Massengil-Beecham (Bristol, Tenn.) |
| Adrenoxyl® | Labaz (Brussels) |
| Afibrin® | Lederle (Buenos Aires) |
| Amicar® | Lederle (USA) |
| Antagosan® | Behring: Hoechst (Frankfurt) |
| Antemovis® | Vister (Milan) |
| Anvitoff® | Knoll (Ludwigshafen) |
| Arhémapectine® | Gallier (Paris) |
| Arwin® | Knoll (Ludwigshafen) |
| Botropase® | Ravizza (Muggiò, Milan) |
| Capillarema® | Baldacci (Pisa) |
| Capracid® | Kabi (Stockholm) |
| Capramol® | Choay (Paris) |
| Caprocid® | Merck Sharp and Dohme (West Point, Pa.) |
| Caprolest® | Pharmachemie (Haarlem) |
| Caprolisin® | Malesci (Florence) |
| Clauden® | Luitpold-Werke (Munich) |
| Coagulen® | Ciba (Varese) |
| Coazimol® | Bruschettini (Genoa) |
| Cyklokapron® | Kabi (Stockholm) |
| Dagynil® | Dagra (Diemen) |
| Defibrase® | Pentapharm (Basle) |
| Dicynene® | Delandale (Canterbury) |
| Dicynone® | Delandale (Canterbury) |
| EACA Roche® | Hoffmann-Laroche (Basle) |
| Eacina® | Zoja (Milan) |
| Ecapron® | Hoechst (Frankfurt) |
| Emex® | Archifar (Milan) |
| Epsikapron® | Kabi (Stockholm) |

| | |
|---|---|
| Epsilon-Tachostyptan® | Hormon-Chemie (Munich) |
| Equigyne® | Merell Toraude (Paris) |
| Exacyl® | Choay (Paris) |
| Frénolyse® | Specia (Paris) |
| Frénovex® | Crinex (Montrouge) |
| Gumbix® | Kali-Chemie (Hannover) |
| H-6102® | Winthrop (New York) |
| Haemostop® | Consolidated Chemicals (Wrexham) |
| Haemostypticum Revici® | Schwarzhaupt (Cologne) |
| Hemocaprol® | Delegrange (Paris) |
| Hemostatique Ercé® | Robert et Carrière (Paris) |
| Iniprol® | Choay (Paris) |
| Karbinone® | Seresci (Brussels) |
| Koagamin® | Chatham (Newark, N.J.) |
| Manetol® | Bayer (Leverkusen) |
| Mediaven® | Medial (Geneva) |
| Naphthionin® | OM Laboratories (Geneva) |
| OM-Dicinona® | OM Laboratories (Geneva) |
| Ophidiase® | Labaz (Bordeaux) |
| Ovestin® | OM Laboratories (Geneva) |
| Premarin® | Ayerst (New York) |
| Presomen® | Kali-Chemie (Hannover) |
| Reptilase® | Pentapharm (Basle) |
| Sangostop® | Endopharm (Frankfurt) |
| Strypturon® | Abbott (North Chicago, Ill.) |
| Styptanon® | Organon (Oss) |
| Styptosolut® | Delta-Pharma (Pfullingen) |
| Tachostyptan® | Hormon-Chemie (Munich) |
| Thrombase® | I.S.H. (Paris) |
| Thrombocytine® | Institut Gentile (Pisa) |
| Trasylol® | Bayer (Leverkusen) |
| Ugurol® | Bayer (Leverkusen) |
| Zymofren® | Specia (Paris) |